Inherited Metabolic Diseases

A guide to 100 conditions

The National Information Centre for
Metabolic Diseases

Edited by

Steve Hannigan

Executive Director

Radcliffe Publishing
Oxford • New York

Radcliffe Publishing Ltd
18 Marcham Road
Abingdon
Oxon OX14 1AA
United Kingdom

www.radcliffe-oxford.com
Electronic catalogue and worldwide online ordering facility.

© 2007 The National Information Centre for Metabolic Diseases

New research and clinical experience can result in changes in treatment and drug therapy. Readers of this book should therefore check the most recent product information on any drug they may prescribe to ensure they are complying with the manufacturer's recommendations concerning dosage, the method and duration of administration, and contraindications. Neither the publisher nor the authors accept liability for any injury or damage arising from this publication.

British Library Cataloguing in Publication Data

A catalogue record for this book is available from the British Library.

ISBN-10 1 84619 099 1
ISBN-13 978 184619 099 5

Typeset by Anne Joshua & Associates, Oxford
Printed and bound by TJI Digital, Padstow, Cornwall

Contents

A note from the Executive Director of Climb   vi
Specialist Advisers   vii
Introduction   x

1 Amino acid disorders and urea cycle disorders   1
Argininosuccinic aciduria   2
Citrullinaemia   4
Hartnup disease   5
Homocystinuria   7
Maple syrup disease   8
Molybdenum cofactor deficiency   10
Non-ketotic hyperglycinaemia   11
Ornithine transcarbamylase deficiency   13
Phenylketonuria   15
Tyrosinaemia type 1   17

2 Organic acid disorders and disorders of fatty acid oxidation   19
Canavan leukodystrophy   20
Carnitine palmitoyltransferase deficiency   22
Glutaric aciduria type 1   24
Isovaleric acidaemia   26
Medium-chain acyl CoA dehydrogenase deficiency   27
Methylglutaconic aciduria (3) – type 2   28
Methylmalonic acidaemia   30
Multiple acyl CoA dehydrogenase deficiency   32
Propionic acidaemia   33
Trimethylaminuria syndrome   35

3 Mitochondrial and peroxisomal disorders   37
Adrenoleukodystrophy – X-linked   38
Alper's disease   40
Fumarase deficiency   42
Kearns–Sayre syndrome   43
Leigh syndrome   44
Mitochondrial encephalopathy, lactic acidosis and stroke-like episodes   46
Mitochondrial respiratory chain complex IV   48
Pearson's syndrome   50
Pyruvate dehydrogenase deficiency   51
Zellweger syndrome   53

4 **Lysosomal, sterol and lipid disorders**   **54**
   Anderson–Fabry disease   55
   Batten disease – infantile form   57
   Cystinosis   58
   Fucosidosis   60
   Gaucher disease type 1   62
   GM2 gangliosidosis type 2 – infantile form   64
   Lipodystrophy – Berardinelli–Seip syndrome   65
   Mucopolysaccharidosis type 2   66
   Niemann–Pick disease – type A   68
   Tay–Sachs disease – infantile form   69

5 **Carbohydrate and glycosylation disorders**   **70**
   Congenital disorders of glycosylation – type Ia   71
   Fanconi–Bickel syndrome   73
   Fructose intolerance – hereditary   74
   Galactosaemia   75
   Glucose transporter type 1 deficiency   77
   Glycogen storage disease type III   78
   Glycogen synthase deficiency   79
   Hyperinsulinism–hypoglycaemia   80
   Sucrase isomaltase deficiency   81
   Uridine diphosphate galactose-4-epimerase deficiency   82

6 **Purine, pyrimidine and porphyria disorders**   **83**
   Acute intermittent porphyria   84
   Adenosine deaminase deficiency   85
   Adenylosuccinate lyase deficiency   86
   Dihydropyrimidine dehydrogenase deficiency   87
   Lesch–Nyhan disease   88
   Myoadenylate deaminase deficiency   90
   Purine nucleoside phosphorylase deficiency   91
   Pyrimidine 5'-nucleotidase deficiency   92
   Variegate porphyria   93
   Xanthine oxidase deficiency   95

7 **Hormone disorders**   **96**
   Pseudohypoaldosteronism type 1   97
   ACTH deficiency   98
   Albright hereditary osteodystrophy   99
   Bannayan–Riley–Ruvalcaba syndrome   101
   Coffin–Siris syndrome   103
   Congenital adrenal hyperplasia – 3-beta-hydroxysteroid dehydrogenase   104
   Growth hormone deficiency   105
   Hypopituitarism   106
   Leprechaunism   107
   Prader–Willi syndrome   108

8   Musculoskeletal disorders and connective tissue disorders   110
    Amyloidosis   111
    Charcot–Marie–Tooth disease   112
    Coffin–Lowry syndrome   114
    Epidermolysis bullosa   116
    Hutchinson–Gilford progeria   118
    Lafora body disease   120
    Lowe syndrome   121
    Russell–Silver syndrome   123
    Velocardiofacial syndrome   124
    X-linked hypophosphataemic rickets   126

9   Blood and immune system disorders   127
    Acrodermatitis enteropathica   128
    Alpha-1-antitrypsin deficiency   129
    Ataxia telangiectasia   131
    Blue rubber bleb naevus syndrome   133
    Factor X deficiency   134
    Gilbert syndrome   135
    Glucose-6-phosphate dehydrogenase deficiency   136
    Turner syndrome   137
    Von Willebrand disease   139
    Wiskott–Aldrich syndrome   141

10 Associated disorders   143
    Bloom syndrome   144
    Cockayne syndrome   145
    Drash syndrome   147
    Hallervorden–Spatz syndrome   148
    Menkes disease   150
    Pelizaeus–Merzbacher disease   151
    Reye syndrome   153
    Smith–Lemli–Opitz syndrome   154
    Timothy syndrome   155
    Xeroderma pigmentosum   157

Index   159

A note from the Executive Director of Climb

I joined Climb in late 2000 after running a respite care charity for four years. Before joining I had never really come across metabolic diseases as a group, but I had heard of a couple of individual diseases. As the Executive Director of Climb and the National Information Centre I am delighted at the support we have received from families and specialists in putting this book together. It will be the first in a series of seven books, which may extend to more when new diseases are identified.

All profits from the publication of this and other books in the series will go directly to the charity and will be used to provide continued support to people affected by metabolic diseases.

Steve Hannigan
Executive Director, Climb
January 2007

Specialist Advisers

The Specialist Advisers who have been involved with this book, and to whom we owe a tremendous debt of gratitude, are listed below.

Dr RA Barker, BA, MBBS, MRCP, PhD
University Lecturer and Honorary Consultant in Neurology, Cambridge Centre for Brain Repair, Cambridge

Professor GT Berry, MD
Professor of Pediatrics and Biochemistry, Jefferson Medical College, Philadelphia, USA

Dr G Besley, BSc, PhD, FRCPCH (Hon)
Head of Laboratory, Willink Biochemical Genetics Unit, Manchester

Dr A Chakrapani, MD, DCH, FRCPCH
Consultant in Inherited Metabolic Disorders, Birmingham Children's Hospital, Birmingham

Mr and Mrs J Chamberlayne
British Porphyria Association (BPA), Durham

Charcot–Marie–Tooth Support Group
Christchurch, UK

Child Growth Foundation
Chiswick, London

Dr M Cleary, MD, MRCPH, MBChB
Consultant Metabolic Paediatrician, Great Ormond Street Hospital, London

Professor T Cox, MA, MSc, MD (Cantab), FRCP, FMedSci
Consultant, Gaucher Disease Team, Addenbrooke's Hospital, Cambridge

Dr CA Davies, PhD
Research Fellow, Division of Laboratory and Regenerative Medicine, University of Manchester, Manchester

Ms J Denyer, RGN, RSCN, RHV
Nurse Consultant in Epidermolysis Bullosa (Paediatric), DebRA

Mrs S Elford
Honorary Chairman, Climb Congenital Adrenal Hyperplasia Support Group

Dr L Fairbanks, PhD
Clinical Scientist, Purine Research Laboratory, Guy's Hospital, London

Dr A Fryer, BSc, MD, FRCP, FRCPCH
Consultant Clinical Geneticist, Alder Hey Hospital, Liverpool

Professor M Gardiner, MD, FRCPCH, FMedSci
Professor of Paediatrics, University College London, London

Ms J Gick, BSc, RSCN
Paediatric Metabolic Nurse Specialist, Guy's Hospital, London

Dr KC Gilmour, PhD
Clinical Scientist – Immunology, Great Ormond Street for Children NHS Trust, London

Dr A Habel, MB ChB, MRCPCH, FRCP
Consultant Paediatrician, Great Ormond Street Hospital, London

Professor PN Hawkins, FRC, FMedSci, PhD, FRCP, MRCP, MBBS
Professor of Medicine and Clinical Director, National Amyloidosis Centre, London

Dr MJ Henderson, BSc, PhD, FRCPath, FRCPCH
Consultant Paediatric Biochemist, St James' University Hospital, Leeds and Director of the Yorkshire Regional Biochemical Genetics Laboratory, Leeds

Dr C Hendriksz, MB ChB, MSc, MRCP, MRCPCH, PG Dip Child Health
Consultant in Clinical Inherited Metabolic Disorders, Birmingham Children's Hospital, Birmingham

Professor ID Hickson, PhD
Professor of Molecular Oncology/Deputy Director, CR-UK Oxford Cancer Centre, Oxford

Dr D Keeling, BSc, MD, FRCP, FRCPath
Consultant Haematologist, Oxford Radcliffe Hospitals, Oxford

Professor DA Kelly, MD, FRCPI, FRCP
Professor of Paediatric Hepatology, Birmingham Children's Hospital, Birmingham

Dr K Lachlan, MB ChB, MRCPCH
Specialist Registrar in Clinical Genetics, Wessex Regional Genetics Service, Southampton

Dr C Lambert, FIBMS, MSc
Section Leader, Red Cell Protein Laboratory, King's College Hospital, London

Professor AR Lehmann, BA, PhD
Chairman, Genome Damage and Stability Centre, University of Sussex, Brighton

Professor J Leonard, MA, MB, BCh PhD, FRCP, FRCPCH
Former Professor of Paediatric Metabolic Disease, Institute of Child Health, London

Lowe Syndrome Trust
London, UK

Dr P McKiernan, BSc, MB, BCh, MRCP (UK), FRCPCH
Consultant Paediatric Hepatologist, Birmingham Children's Hospital, Birmingham

Dr MA McShane, MB, BCh, MRCP(UK)
Consultant Paediatric Neurologist, John Radcliffe Hospital, Oxford

Dr A Morris, BM, BCh, MA, PhD, FRCPCH
Consultant Paediatrician with Special Interest in Inherited Metabolic Diseases, Willink Biochemical Unit, Manchester Children's Hospital

Dr Z Mughal, MB, ChB, FRCP, FRCPCH, DCH
Consultant Paediatrician and Honorary Senior Lecturer in Child Health, St Mary's Hospital for Women and Children, Manchester

Dr RE Pugh, MB, ChB, FRCP, FRCPCH
Consultant Paediatrician, Mid Cheshire Hospital Trust, Crewe

Dr S Rahman, BM, BCh, MRCP, PhD
Clinical Lecturer in Paediatric Metabolic Medicine, Institute of Child Health, University College London and Great Ormond Street Hospital, London

Dr U Ramaswami, MD, MSc, FRCPCH
Consultant Metabolic Paediatrician, Addenbrooke's Hospital, Cambridge

Dr PH Robinson, BSc, MB, BCh, MRCP (UK), FRCPCH
Consultant in Paediatric Metabolic Disease, Royal Hospital for Sick Children, Glasgow

Dr A Simmonds, MSc, PhD, Dip Chem Path
Emeritus Senior Lecturer, Purine Research Unit, Guy's Hospital, London

Dr R Stanhope, BSc, MD, DCH, FRCP, FRCPCH
Consultant Paediatric Endocrinologist, Institute of Child Health, London

Dr C Steward, MA, BM, BCh, PhD, FRCPCH, FRCP
Honorary Consultant in Bone Marrow Transplantation for Genetic Diseases, Bristol Royal Hospital for Sick Children, Bristol

Professor PM Stewart, MD, FDRCP, FMedSci
Professor of Medicine, University of Birmingham, Birmingham

Professor JG Thoene, MD
Director, Hayward Genetics Center, New Orleans, USA

Dr JH Walter, MD, FRCPCH
Consultant Paediatrician, Willink Biochemical Unit, Manchester Children's Hospital, Manchester

Professor J Wass, MA, MD, FRCP
Professor of Endocrinology, Nuffield Orthopaedic Centre, Oxford

Dr M Webster, MB, ChB, FRCP, FRCPCH, DCH
Consultant Paediatrician, Taunton and Somerset Hospital, Taunton

Introduction

About Climb

Children Living with Inherited Metabolic Diseases (Climb) is a registered charity in the UK, and as an organisation we see many books whose subject is one of the many metabolic diseases. We currently support over 700 of these diseases, and the majority of our information is presented in a family-friendly format which, I am sorry to say, cannot be said about a lot of the information that is available in published form or on the Internet.

The charity was started in 1981 and changed its name to Climb in 1999. In 2004 we launched the National Information Centre for Metabolic Diseases as part of the Climb group. Since the launch of the National Information Centre our support base has grown considerably, and in 2005–06 we provided information and support to over 23,000 families and professionals worldwide, and supported individuals and organisations in over 80 different countries.

This is the first of several books designed as a guide for anyone affected by or working with metabolic diseases. Through this medium we are trying to help people to understand, in a family-friendly way, what the particular disease involves. We have divided the 700 diseases that we support into 10 main groups, which are as follows:

- amino acid and urea cycle disorders
- organic acid and fatty acid oxidation disorders
- mitochondrial and peroxisomal disorders
- lysosomal, sterol and lipid disorders
- carbohydrate and glycosylation disorders
- purine, pyrimidine and porphyria disorders
- hormone disorders
- musculoskeletal and connective tissue disorders
- blood and immune system disorders
- associated disorders.

In this, the first volume, we have covered 100 diseases, ranging from those that affect approximately 1 in 10,000 people to diseases that are very rare and affect around 1 in 100,000.

We update our information on a regular basis, and we work with a large group of Specialist Advisers around the world to ensure that the information is correct and up to date.

The idea for the books came from our Executive Director, Steve Hannigan, and the trustees and staff have been very supportive in the production of the information contained in this book. Our Information Research Officer, Helen Watts, deserves a special mention, as her dedication, tact and diplomacy as the liaison for our Specialist Advisers have been pivotal in the gathering of information for publication.

Metabolic diseases

Each of the different metabolic diseases is inherited through one of four routes. These are summarised below.

Autosomal dominant inheritance

This method of inheritance occurs when a single copy of the diseased gene will dominate the other normal gene. Therefore if a defective gene is inherited from either parent, the child will be affected with the disorder. This means that for each pregnancy if either of the parents has a defective gene, there is a 50% chance of a child being affected by the disease.

Autosomal recessive inheritance

This occurs when a child inherits a gene for the disease from both parents. The risk that the offspring of a couple who are both carriers of the disease will be affected is 25%. There is a 50% chance that their child will be a carrier, and there is a 25% chance that the child will not carry the abnormal gene.

MtDNA inheritance

Disorders inherited in this way are caused by a defect in the mitochondrial DNA (mtDNA). This can be inherited from the maternal line, as the mtDNA is only passed down from mothers to their children. During fertilisation the instructions in the mtDNA from the father are lost, so all the instructions in the mtDNA come from the mother. This means that girls will always pass on a defect in their mtDNA and boys will never pass on a defect in their mtDNA to their children.

X-linked inheritance

This occurs when diseases are coded on the X chromosomes of genes. Females have two X chromosomes, and any disease trait on one of the X chromosomes is usually masked by the other normal X chromosome. Males have one X and one Y chromosome, so because there is only one X chromosome, 50% of male children may inherit the disease.

Chapter 1

Amino acid disorders and urea cycle disorders

Amino acid disorders

Amino acid disorders can be caused by problems with transport of the amino acids into the cells or by impairment of the breakdown of amino acids. Amino acids are the building blocks of proteins. Some amino acids can be synthesised by the body, while others must be obtained through protein from the diet. The latter are known as the essential amino acids. A deficiency in one of the enzymes needed to break down amino acids means that the body is unable to use them for growth and repair. Newborn babies are routinely screened for several metabolic disorders. Of these screening tests, the most commonly known is the heel prick test, which is used to diagnose phenylketonuria (PKU).

Urea cycle disorders

The urea cycle disorders (UCDs) are a group of genetic disorders that are caused by a deficiency of one of six enzymes in the urea cycle, which is responsible for the removal of ammonia. These six enzymes are:

- arginase
- argininosuccinate lyase
- argininosuccinate synthetase
- carbamyl phosphate synthetase
- N-acetylglutamate synthetase
- ornithine transcarbamylase.

When protein is digested by the body, it is broken down into small molecules known as amino acids. These are transported via the bloodstream to the cells. They may be used to build bodily protein or to produce glucose and energy. Most of us eat more protein than we need to, and the excess amino acids are converted to ammonia, which is a toxic substance. In the liver the ammonia is converted into a harmless substance known as urea, which is excreted in the urine. In UCDs, the functioning of one of the six enzymes is impaired and ammonia is not removed from the bloodstream. This leads to a build-up of ammonia with high blood concentrations (hyper-ammonaemia), causing the symptoms of these disorders.

Argininosuccinic aciduria

Other names for this condition

- Argininosuccinase deficiency
- Argininosuccinate lyase deficiency
- Argininosuccinic acidaemia
- ASA
- ASL

This disorder is one of a group of conditions, known as the urea cycle disorders, in which the body's ability to manage dietary protein is impaired. In argininosuccinic aciduria there is a deficiency or absence of the enzyme argininosuccinate lyase (ASL), which is an important part of the urea cycle. This leads to an accumulation of the amino acid argininosuccinic acid (hence the name), and may lead to a build-up of ammonia (and its related product glutamine) in the body, giving rise to the symptoms of the disorder.

The pattern of inheritance of this disorder is autosomal recessive. It is thought to occur in about 1 in 70,000 of the population.

Like many inherited metabolic diseases, argininosuccinic aciduria may manifest itself at different ages and in different ways. This probably depends on whether the enzyme is completely or partially absent. In the severe form of ASA, babies show complete absence of the ASL enzyme and exhibit symptoms soon after birth. There is usually a symptom-free period of 24–48 hours with normal feeding, before the baby becomes lethargic, with poor feeding, vomiting, irritability and liver enlargement (hepatomegaly). These symptoms are similar to, and often mistaken for, those of infection. As the ammonia level rises, breathing problems (apnoea), seizures and coma may ensue, with swelling of the brain (cerebral oedema). If left untreated, this severe form is life-threatening. Even with appropriate treatment, the baby may suffer significant neurological impairment or may not survive.

Partial deficiency of the ASL enzyme leads to a less severe form of ASA in which symptoms may not develop until infancy or childhood. Typically they may appear at the time of weaning or change from formula to cows' milk. Infection or high protein intake may also precipitate symptoms. These may include recurrent acute episodes of vomiting, lethargy, sleepiness, agitation, seizures and coma, or a more gradual failure to gain weight and delay in neurological development. Children with ASL may develop movement disorders (ataxia) and an aversion to higher-protein foods. Characteristically the hair is brittle and remains short.

Even in the milder forms of ASL, high levels of ammonia during acute episodes may affect the brain and lead to long-term neurological impairment.

In the acute situation with very high ammonia levels (severe hyperammonaemic episodes), it is important to reduce the ammonia levels as quickly as possible. Intravenous drugs (arginine, sodium benzoate and phenylbutyrate) help to boost the effectiveness of the urea cycle and enable the excretion of ammonia in the urine by using different metabolic pathways. Protein intake is temporarily stopped and intravenous glucose is given to provide energy and to reduce the breakdown of bodily protein (catabolism). Haemodialysis (blood filtering by machine) may be necessary to remove ammonia directly from the bloodstream.

The aim of long-term treatment is to reduce the accumulation of ammonia and to try to avoid acute hyperammonaemic episodes. There are three main components to the treatment, which should be undertaken with the help of a metabolic team.

First, dietary protein intake is restricted in order to limit the amount of ammonia that the urea cycle has to deal with. This includes the substitution of familiar foods such as pasta, rice and flour with low-protein alternatives, and usually the addition of essential amino acid mixtures, multivitamins and calcium. Secondly, oral medication (arginine, sodium benzoate and phenylbutyrate) given through the day acts in the same way as in the acute episodes. In some children this medication is most easily given through a gastrostomy tube (a tube that is placed in the stomach through the abdominal wall) or a nasogastric tube (a tube that passes through the nose and into the stomach). The effectiveness of this treatment is monitored by regular blood tests and assessment of growth, and diet and drug doses are adjusted as necessary. Thirdly, an emergency regime of high-glucose, zero-protein drinks is used when the child becomes unwell. This is often enough to enable short illnesses to be managed at home.

Liver transplantation has been used in some severe cases of this disorder.

Reviewed by Dr M Webster

Citrullinaemia

Other names for this condition
- ASS deficiency
- Argininosuccinate synthetase deficiency
- Citrullinuria
- Inborn error of urea synthesis, citrullinaemia type I
- Urea cycle disorder, citrullinaemia type I

Citrullinaemia belongs to a group of six disorders known as the urea cycle disorders. In this particular disorder there is a deficiency or absence of the enzyme argininosuccinate synthetase, and consequently ammonia is not converted into urea.

This disorder is genetically inherited from the parents in an autosomal recessive fashion.

The severity of the disorder and the age of onset vary from one individual to another. Individuals who have a severe form of citrullinaemia often present with symptoms soon after birth. These can include refusal to feed, vomiting, lethargy, irritability, a lack of muscle tone (hypotonia), an enlarged liver (hepatomegaly), breathing difficulties, seizures and the accumulation of fluid in the brain (cerebral oedema). Individuals with this disorder may progress to coma due to high ammonia levels in the blood.

Individuals with milder forms of the disorder, who have only a partial deficiency of the enzyme, may not develop symptoms until infancy or childhood. Symptoms in these children are highly variable and may include vomiting, poor appetite, poor developmental progress, episodes of lethargy, and ataxia, among many others. If left untreated, symptoms can lead to coma. Often in children the symptoms are episodic and may be associated with fasting or an infection as the body breaks down stored proteins. In some cases coma may occur.

Treatment of an acute episode includes restriction of any further intake of protein. Glucose is usually given to reduce the breakdown of any protein, as this would increase ammonia levels further. Medication (arginine, sodium benzoate and sodium phenylbutyrate) is used to bring the ammonia levels down, and if body levels are very high, dialysis may be needed to help to reduce them. Aggressive treatment is needed for hyperammonaemic episodes that have progressed to loss of consciousness.

Long-term treatment aims to prevent the accumulation of high levels of ammonia in the body with a low-protein diet and medication.

Reviewed by Professor J Leonard

Hartnup disease

Other names for this condition
- Hartnup disorder
- Hartnup syndrome
- Hart syndrome
- H disease
- HND
- Pellagra–cerebellar ataxia–renal aminoaciduria syndrome
- Tryptophan pyrrolase deficiency

Hartnup disease is a rare disorder caused by an inborn error of amino acid metabolism. A defect in tryptophan, an amino acid essential for nutrition, impairs the body's ability to break down and transport amino acids through the intestines. Hartnup disease is caused by a defective gene which has been located on the long arm of chromosome 11. In some cases the defective gene may be found on the short arm of chromosome 5. This gene is known as the SLC9A19 gene, and it encodes transport of sodium-dependent amino acids.

Hartnup disease is genetically inherited from the parents in an autosomal recessive fashion.

Symptoms of the disease vary from case to case, and many individuals do not show any symptoms. When symptoms do occur, the most common characteristics are an intolerance of light, causing red, scaly rashes on the face and hands and any other parts of the body that are exposed to the light. Acute attacks of this disorder may be caused by exposure to sunlight, sulphonamide medications, stress and/or poor nutrition, and the frequency of attacks usually decreases with age. Symptoms include poor coordination, unsteadiness when walking (gait), muscle coordination difficulties (ataxia), speech problems, problems with the stomach and intestines, vertigo, and tremors in the hands and tongue. Affected individuals may have visual difficulties such as double vision (diplopia), involuntary eye movements (nystagmus), squinting and droopiness of the eyelids. Those affected may also have neurological problems, such as mild learning difficulties, developmental delay, behavioural problems, impaired intellectual abilities (dementia), emotional instability and depression. Delusions or hallucinations may also be apparent. Diarrhoea and fainting are common in individuals affected by Hartnup disease, and other symptoms include short stature, seizures, persistent headaches and low muscle tone (hypotonia). Mild heart irregularities may be apparent, but this symptom is extremely rare. Those affected may also have abnormal levels of amino acids in the urine (aminoaciduria).

Hartnup disease may be diagnosed by the presence of a unique pattern of amino acids in the urine. This may be ascertained by urine tests performed during routine screening at birth. Diet plays a major role in the treatment of this condition, so good nutrition must be maintained. Affected individuals should avoid sunlight and sulphonamide drugs, and should take nicotinamide or niacin supplements. Treatment may also include supplements of an oral drug called L-tryptophan ethyl. Genetic counselling may be of benefit to those affected by this condition.

Reviewed by Dr RE Pugh

Homocystinuria

This disorder belongs to a group of conditions known as the amino acid disorders, in which there is an absence or deficiency of an enzyme that is needed to break down proteins into amino acids, which prevents the body from using proteins for growth and repair. The amino acid methionine is converted into homocysteine, which is in turn converted into cysteine. In homocystinuria there is a deficiency or absence of an enzyme called cystathionine beta-synthase (CBS), which is required to break down homocysteine into cysteine. This leads to a build-up of homocysteine in the body, especially in the blood (homocysteinaemia) and the urine (homocystinuria). In addition, there are increased levels of methionine.

This disorder is genetically inherited from the parents in an autosomal recessive fashion.

There are other forms of homocystinuria that are caused by the following enzyme deficiencies:

- methylene tetrahydrofolate reductase deficiency
- a defect in either cobalamin E or cobalamin G that causes methylcobalamin deficiency
- a defect in either cobalamin C, cobalamin D or cobalamin F that causes a deficiency in both adenosylcobalamin and methylcobalamin, leading to combined methylmalonic acidaemia and homocystinuria.

Symptoms of homocystinuria usually include a delay in physical development, seizures and long-term flushing of the face. In addition, there can be dislocation of the lens of the eye, as well as short-sightedness and increased pressure within the eye (glaucoma). Individuals with this condition tend to be tall, with long limbs and fingers. Those affected may also have chest and/or knee deformities, and there may be thinning and weakening of the bones (osteoporosis) which can lead to frequent fractures and restricted joint mobility. Individuals are prone to the formation of blood clots in veins and arteries, which can lead to stroke and blockage of these vessels anywhere in the body. Other symptoms include mild learning difficulties, a high narrow palate and an enlarged liver.

Homocystinuria can be diagnosed by means of urine tests that demonstrate high levels of cysteine in the urine. Other tests may include analysis of methionine, homocysteine and cystathionine levels in the urine, and a liver biopsy and/or skin biopsy to measure enzyme activity. This disorder can also be diagnosed by newborn screening programmes. In some individuals, treatment of this disorder includes giving large doses of vitamin B_6 (pyridoxine), which helps to convert homocysteine into cysteine. Other individuals do not respond to this supplement, in which case the condition is best controlled by diet. This involves restricting intake of the amino acid methionine and giving cysteine supplements. In addition, vitamin B_{12}, folic acid and betaine may be of benefit. Other medication can help to relieve symptoms. It is advised that affected individuals do not use oral contraceptives.

Reviewed by Dr G Besley

Maple syrup disease

Other names for this condition
- BCKD deficiency
- Branched-chain alpha-ketoacid dehydrogenase deficiency
- Maple syrup urine disease
- MSUD
- MSD

This is a rare inherited metabolic disease that is characterised by an unusual odour of the urine, sweat and ear wax. Symptoms occur because the body is unable to break down three amino acids, namely leucine, isoleucine and valine, due to a deficiency of the enzyme necessary for this breakdown. This leads to an increase in these amino acids in the blood that reaches toxic levels, and can lead to damage to the body tissues, including the brain. There is wide variation in the severity of the disease. Individuals with the most severe form of the disease develop symptoms soon after birth, whereas the milder form may present in later childhood.

This condition is genetically inherited from the parents in an autosomal recessive fashion.

There are different forms of maple syrup disease, which vary in severity and in the extent of enzyme deficiency. The lower the enzyme activity, the more severe the symptoms.

- The classical form of the disease has very low enzyme activity. Symptoms develop in newborns within days of birth, and include a sweet odour of the urine, sweat and ear wax, poor feeding, vomiting, breathing irregularities, episodes of muscle rigidity (hypertonia) with contrasting episodes of floppiness (hypotonia), lethargy, high levels of acid in the blood (metabolic acidosis), seizures and coma. Learning difficulties and behavioural problems may be apparent in older children.
- In the intermediate form there is normally enzyme activity that is approximately 3–8% of normal levels. Symptoms usually develop within the first few months of life, when the child is ill or fasting. The symptoms are the same as those that occur in the classical form, but usually milder.
- In the intermittent form there is normally enzyme activity that is approximately 8–15% of normal levels. In this form, the disorder usually presents even later in childhood. These children are normally healthy, but symptoms are brought on by an infection, fasting or surgery. The symptoms are similar to those that occur in the classical form, and affected individuals may also be unable to coordinate voluntary movements (ataxia).
- Children with the thiamine-responsive form have mild or occasional symptoms, which improve when thiamine is given. This is because in this form the thiamine increases the activity of the missing enzyme. This form is very rare.

Maple syrup disease can be diagnosed in newborn screening programmes that are performed routinely in order to identify a number of metabolic conditions. It is not routine to test for maple syrup disease in the UK. Blood tests are used to confirm the diagnosis.

Once this condition has been diagnosed, treatment should begin as soon as possible following birth, as it can reduce the severity of the symptoms. There are two main strategies for treatment. Firstly, a high-energy diet can be given that does not include the amino acids affected by the metabolic block (leucine, isoleucine and valine) if there is an excessive accumulation of acid in the body (metabolic acidosis). Secondly, toxins can be removed from the blood by administering special fluids (dialysis) through the abdominal wall. Affected individuals should be placed on a diet that does not include high-protein foods such as meat, fish, nuts, eggs, dairy and soya produce. The supplementation of calories and a special formula are usually required to ensure that the child receives all the other proteins necessary for growth and development. The diet is strict and compliance is not easy. A special plan needs to be followed during the ongoing illness of children, in order to prevent serious complications. Individuals with the thyamine-responsive form of the disease are treated with large doses of thiamine in the newborn period.

Reviewed by Professor J Leonard

Molybdenum cofactor deficiency

Other names for this condition
- MOCOD
- Sulphite and xanthine oxidase deficiency
- Sulphite oxidase, xanthine dehydrogenase and aldehyde oxidase combined deficiency

In this disorder there is a deficiency of three enzymes. This is because molybdenum is required in three different enzymes, namely sulphite oxidase, xanthine oxidase and aldehyde oxidase, which catalyse three different processes:

1. the conversion of sulphite to sulphate by sulphite oxidase, which is involved in the breakdown of sulphur-containing proteins (amino acids)
2. the conversion of xanthine to uric acid by xanthine oxidase, which is important in uric acid formation and aids the transort of iron from the liver for use around the body
3. the conversion of aldehydes to acids by aldehyde oxidase, which forms part of the processing of carbohydrates and alcohol.

This disorder is genetically inherited from the parents in an autosomal recessive fashion.

Most individuals who present with this disorder do so shortly after birth. Common symptoms include seizures that are resistant to medication, feeding difficulties, loss of muscle tone (hypotonia), a small-sized head (microcephaly), delays in mental development, increased levels of taurine, *S*-sulphocysteine and thiosulphate and xanthine in the urine, and low levels of uric acid in the blood (hypouricaemia) and urine (uricaciduria). In some cases there may also be increased sulphite levels in the urine. Specific spasms that cause the head and the heel to bend backwards while the body is bent over (opisthotonos) may occur. Individuals often have characteristic facial features such as deep-set eyes and a depressed nasal bridge, and there can be malformations in the brain structure. Dislocation of the lens of the eye frequently occurs in the first two years, and can lead to blurring of the vision. Occasionally, some individuals present with a partial deficiency of molybdenum cofactor in childhood. These individuals show a loss of muscle tone (hypotonia), lens dislocation and loss of previously acquired skills.

Treatment of this disease aims to relieve any symptoms and support the care of the individual. Those who first show symptoms during the neonatal period rarely survive beyond late infancy. There have been isolated case reports of individuals with the later-onset form showing some improvement in response to restricted dietary intake of sulphur-containing amino acids.

Reviewed by Dr MJ Henderson

Non-ketotic hyperglycinaemia

Other names for this condition
- Glycine encephalopathy
- NKH
- Non-ketotic glycinaemia

In this disorder, affected individuals are unable to break down a specific amino acid, glycine, into smaller molecules. This means that there is a build-up of large amounts of this amino acid in the body, especially in the blood, the urine and the cerebrospinal fluid (CSF, the fluid that surrounds the spinal cord and the brain). This accumulation of glycine leads to the symptoms of the disorder, which can include seizures and delayed development.

This disorder is genetically inherited from the parents in an autosomal recessive fashion.

There are four forms of non-ketotic hyperglycinaemia.

1 The neonatal form presents in the first few days of life, generally after the first feed has occurred, which will have contain the amino acid glycine. Symptoms include a failure to gain weight and grow (failure to thrive), a lack of muscle tone (hypotonia), a weak cry, drowsiness and lethargy, which can progress to a comatose state. Seizures are also common in this disorder. There is usually an associated delay in development due to the toxic accumulation of glycine. Children with this disease will be seriously ill, and few survive the neonatal period. Those who do survive usually show serious delay in cognitive development.

2 The infantile form usually presents after approximately 6 months. Symptoms include seizures and a delay in physical and mental development, including learning difficulties and behavioural problems.

3 The late-onset form of this disorder presents during childhood. Symptoms include stiffness in both legs, which becomes worse with time (spastic diplegia), and the deterioration of the optic nerve, which leads to blindness.

4 The mild-episodic form generally presents in childhood. Symptoms occur during episodes in which the individual may become delirious and show signs of fever. Affected individuals may make involuntary jerky movements (chorea) and may be unable to look upwards. They may also have mild learning difficulties and behavioural problems.

This disorder is diagnosed by means of laboratory tests to determine the levels of glycine in the blood and CSF. The diagnosis can also be confirmed by proton magnetic resonance spectroscopy, or by direct enzyme assay. A metabolic specialist must be consulted to ensure the correct diagnosis and treatment. Prenatal diagnosis is available. Treatment for seizures may include strychnine (a glycine antagonist), dextromethorphan, ketamine, diazepam and sodium benzoate, with or without choline, and folic acid may also be beneficial. Other treatment is symptomatic and supportive. Research into the use of enzyme replacement therapy to treat this disorder is ongoing.

Reviewed by Professor JG Thoene

Ornithine transcarbamylase deficiency

Other names for this condition
- Hyperammonaemia type II
- Hyperammonaemia due to ornithine transcarbamylase deficiency
- OTC deficiency
- Ornithine carbamoyl transferase deficiency

This disorder belongs to a group of conditions known as the urea cycle disorders. It is characterised by a deficiency or absence of the enzyme ornithine transcarbamylase. As a result, the conversion of ammonia to urea is prevented, leading to a build-up of ammonia in the body (hyperammonaemia), which causes the symptoms of this disorder.

This disorder is genetically inherited from the mother by X-linked inheritance.

The severity of the disorder and the age of onset vary from one individual to another. Those who have a severe form of OTC deficiency show symptoms soon after birth. These can include refusal to feed, vomiting, increasing lethargy, irritability, a lack of muscle tone (hypotonia), an enlarged liver (hepatomegaly), breathing problems, seizures, the accumulation of water in the brain, and possibly coma.

Individuals with milder forms of the disorder, in which there may be a partial deficiency of the enzyme, may not develop symptoms until infancy or childhood. The symptoms that occur in these cases may include hyperactivity or behavioural problems, vomiting, lethargy, confusion, irritability and inability to coordinate movements (ataxia). If left untreated, this condition can lead to coma. In children, an initial episode or further acute episodes may often occur due to a period of fasting or an illness, as the body breaks down stored proteins.

High levels of ammonia in the body can lead to coma, and affected individuals can develop neurological problems such as a delay in mental and physical development, and cerebral palsy.

Treatment of an acute episode includes restriction of any further intake of protein in order to prevent any additional increase in ammonia levels. Affected individuals are placed on a low-protein, high-calorie diet with amino acid supplements. This can be achieved by using special food formulas. Glucose is usually given to prevent the breakdown of any stored protein that would increase ammonia levels further. If ammonia levels are extremely high, medication and possibly dialysis may be needed to help to reduce them. Prompt and aggressive treatment is needed during episodes of high ammonia levels or increased lethargy and severe vomiting.

Medications may also be given to help to remove excess nitrogen from the body. These are used to provide the urea cycle with an alternative means of removing waste nitrogen from the body, and they are administered through a nasogastric tube or a gastrostomy tube. Individuals may also benefit from arginine or citrulline supplements. In addition, multivitamins and calcium supplements may be used in the treatment of this disorder.

Blood tests must be performed on a regular basis to detect any increase in ammonia levels.

Research into this disorder is ongoing.

Reviewed by Dr G Besley

Phenylketonuria

Other names for this condition
- Classical phenylketonuria
- Hyperphenylalaninaemia
- Phenylalanine hydroxylase deficiency
- Phenylalaninaemia
- PKU

In this disorder there is a deficiency or absence of the liver enzyme phenylalanine hydroxylase. This enzyme is needed to break down the amino acid phenylalanine, so its deficiency or absence leads to a build-up of phenylalanine in the brain, which causes profound mental retardation. In most developed countries phenylketonuria (PKU) is tested for at birth.

This disorder is genetically inherited from the parents in an autosomal recessive fashion.

If PKU is not diagnosed by a routine neonatal screening programme, symptoms appear during the first few weeks of life, and usually include vomiting, irritability, abnormal drowsiness and lethargy, as well as feeding difficulties. Affected individuals may also have an unusual musty odour. As the phenylalanine levels increase, a rash similar to eczema, that causes itching, redness and blistering, can develop. Neuro-logical symptoms are also present in some individuals with PKU, and they can vary greatly. There may be jerky muscle movements, abnormally tight muscles (hyper-tonicity), hyperactivity, poor coordination of muscle movements (ataxia), and fits (seizures).

If left untreated, this disorder causes a severe permanent delay in mental develop-ment (with an average IQ of 20), as well as behavioural difficulties.

PKU is treated with a phenylalanine-restricted diet. Phenylalanine occurs in most natural proteins, so these must be avoided and therefore a low-protein diet is needed. Foods high in protein, such as meat, milk, fish and cheese, are typically not allowed. Foods low in protein, such as fruits, vegetables and some cereals, are permitted but only in limited amounts. There are specially prepared food products available that are phenylalanine-free and are of great benefit. However, it is impossible to eliminate protein from the diet altogether without compromising health, as some protein intake is essential for growth and repair of tissues. There are special formulas available that contain all of the essential amino acids except for phenylalanine. Consultation with a metabolic specialist and a metabolic nutritionist is essential in order to maintain the correct amount of phenylalanine in the diet as the child grows. The blood phenyla-lanine concentration must be checked weekly during the first weeks of life, in order to determine the infant's individual tolerance, and thereafter must be checked monthly for life.

When female patients with PKU become pregnant there must be stringent regulation of their dietary phenylalanine intake in order to avoid the devastating effects of elevated maternal phenylalanine levels on the fetus. If maternal phenylalanine levels are properly monitored and controlled, these women can give birth to healthy infants.

Reviewed by Professor JG Thoene

Tyrosinaemia type 1

Other names for this condition
- Congenital tyrosinosis
- Fumarylacetoacetase deficiency
- Hepatorenal tyrosinaemia
- Hereditary tyrosinaemia type 1

Tyrosinaemia type 1 is a rare metabolic disorder characterised by raised levels of the amino acid tyrosine in the blood. The disorder occurs when there is an absence or deficiency of an enzyme known as fumarylacetoacetate hydrolase, which is needed to break down tyrosine. If this amino acid is not broken down, it accumulates in the body, especially in the liver, kidneys and brain. Individuals may present with either an acute or a chronic form of this condition. The two forms are based on the age of the child and the severity of their symptoms.

This disorder is genetically inherited from the parents in an autosomal recessive fashion.

Symptoms vary widely from one case to another. The acute form is present at birth or during the first few weeks of life. Symptoms may include failure to grow and gain weight (failure to thrive), lethargy, irritability, fever, diarrhoea, bloody stools (melaena), vomiting, bruising easily, an enlarged liver (hepatomegaly) and yellowing of the skin (jaundice). Affected individuals may sometimes have a cabbage-like odour. Symptoms can progress to an enlarged spleen (splenomegaly), the accumulation of fluid in the abdomen (ascites), blood-clotting problems, and progressive scarring and impaired function of the liver that can lead to chronic liver failure.

The chronic form of the disorder occurs less frequently, has a more gradual onset, and the symptoms are usually less severe. Symptoms commonly present after the first year with failure to grow and gain weight (failure to thrive) and a delay in physical and mental development. Individuals with the chronic form may eventually develop progressive scarring of the liver (cirrhosis) leading to chronic liver failure, problems with the nerves (polyneuropathy), high blood pressure (hypertension), enlargement and weakening of the heart (hypertrophic cardiomyopathy), and an increased susceptibility to a form of liver cancer known as hepatocellular carcinoma. In addition, individuals may develop renal Fanconi syndrome, which can cause kidney dysfunction, vomiting, dehydration, softening and weakening of the bones (rickets), and fever.

Tyrosinaemia is diagnosed on the basis of a range of specialised tests, a clinical evaluation and family history. The diagnosis can be confirmed by demonstrating the presence of succinylacetone in the urine and decreased activity of the enzyme fumarylacetoacetate hydrolase in liver tissue or cultured fibroblasts. Prenatal diagnosis can be made by measuring the activity of this enzyme in amniotic fluid cells. Some states in the USA test for tyrosinaemia type 1 in the newborn screening programme. Treatment of the disorder includes restricting dietary intake of the amino acids tyrosine and phenylalanine. As these occur in most natural proteins, a low-protein diet is needed. As some protein is essential for normal growth and repair of tissues, specially prepared formulas are required. These contain all of the essential amino acids except tyrosine and phenylalanine. With progression of the condition there may be liver failure that requires a liver transplant. In some cases a transplant can improve the function of the kidneys as well as normalising liver activity. A new drug, NTBC (Nitisinone®), has been developed which blocks the formation of the toxic substances that build up in tyrosinaemia, and improvements in the liver and kidney function of affected individuals have been observed. However, children who are receiving this drug need to be monitored carefully, with frequent follow-up.

Reviewed by Professor JG Thoene

Chapter 2

Organic acid disorders and disorders of fatty acid oxidation

Organic acid disorders

Organic acid disorders are caused by an absence or a deficiency of one or more of the enzymes needed to complete the breakdown of dietary protein. Because the protein cannot be broken down, the body is unable to use it for growth and repair, and there is a build-up of harmful substances, usually acids, in the blood and urine.

Fatty acid oxidation disorders

Fatty acid oxidation disorders (FODs) are caused by an absence or a deficiency of one of several enzymes that are needed to convert stored fats into energy. This means that if the body runs out of its primary source of energy, namely glucose, the fats that would normally be broken down to provide energy are not available. Because of this, long periods without food can lead to severe complications. The commonest fatty acid oxidation disorder is caused by a deficiency of medium-chain acyl CoA dehydrogenase.

Canavan leukodystrophy

Other names for this condition

- ACY2 deficiency
- Aminoacylase-2 deficiency
- Aspartoacylase deficiency
- ASP deficiency
- ASPA deficiency
- CD
- Canavan's disease
- Canavan–Van Bogaert–Bertrand disease
- Spongy degeneration of the central nervous system
- Spongy degeneration of the neuroaxis
- Van Bogaert–Bertrand syndrome

Canavan leukodystrophy is a rare progressive neurological disorder that is caused by a defect in the ASPA gene. This defect leads to a deficiency of the enzyme aspartoacylase, which is responsible for the breakdown of N-acetylaspartic acid, a chemical that is essential for the correct functioning of the brain. The aspartoacylase deficiency leads to deterioration of the central nervous system (the brain and spinal cord), which is the main characteristic of the disorder. Canavan leukodystrophy has a higher prevalence in families of Eastern European Jewish ancestry.

This disorder is genetically inherited from the parents in an autosomal recessive fashion.

Canavan leukodystrophy usually presents between 3 and 5 months of age. The disorder is generally recognised when the child loses previously acquired skills or fails to achieve early milestones. Affected individuals show a progressive mental and physical decline, which is apparent in early infancy. Symptoms may include a loss of muscle tone, irritability, unresponsiveness, and inability to sit, stand, walk and/or talk. The head may be abnormally large (macrocephaly) due to the brain swelling and the bones of the skull not being able to fuse properly. Involuntary muscle contractions in the arms and legs, exaggerated reflexes (hyperreflexia), paralysis and weak neck muscles may become apparent as the disease progresses. Other symptoms include fever, vomiting, sweating, excessive thirst, increased susceptibility to infections, and visual impairment due to deterioration of the optic nerve fibres (optic atrophy). Affected individuals may have life-threatening complications in the first few years of life or later, and rarely survive beyond adolescence. As the child gets older, they may experience sleeping difficulties, feeding problems and seizures.

This disorder can be diagnosed by using gas chromatography–mass spectrometry (GC–MS) to measure the level of N-acetylaspartic acid in the urine. Gene analysis can also confirm the diagnosis. Prenatal diagnosis can be made by testing the level of N-acetylaspartic acid in the amniotic fluid. Chorionic villus sampling (CVS) is available if both parents are known to have the defective gene.

Treatment of Canavan leukodystrophy aims to relieve any symptoms and to provide support with the care of the individual. Physiotherapy may be of benefit to aid mobility, feeding tubes may be used if the individual has difficulty feeding or swallowing, and anti-epileptic drugs may be used for the treatment of seizures. Research into the use of gene therapy and other treatments for this disorder is ongoing.

Reviewed by Dr A Chakrapani

Carnitine palmitoyltransferase deficiency

Other names for this condition
- CPT deficiency
- CPTD
- Myopathy with deficiency of carnitine palmitoyltransferase
- Myopathy – metabolic, carnitine palmitoyltransferase

This disorder is one of a group of conditions known as fatty acid oxidation disorders, where there is a deficiency of a mitochondrial enzyme. Mitochondria are present in every cell in the body, and they produce most of the body's energy to allow movement of muscles, including the heart muscle. The body uses glucose as an energy source, but when this is no longer available, the body breaks down fatty acids in order to obtain energy. In this disorder, due to the deficiency of the enzyme carnitine palmitoyltransferase it is difficult to break down fatty acids to produce energy. Symptoms of the disorder may be triggered by prolonged exercise, and also in some cases by illness, stress, cold and menstruation.

This disorder is genetically inherited from the parents in an autosomal recessive fashion.

There are two types of carnitine palmitoyltransferase deficiency.

- Type 1 usually affects adults and adolescents.
- Type 2 can affect adults, but a severe form of this disorder affects infants.

Both types have the same common symptoms, which may occur in episodes after strenuous exercise, and can include disabling fatigue, muscle pain, muscle stiffness and muscle weakness that may last for days at a time. This can lead to the breakdown of muscles (rhabdomyolysis) and the presence of myoglobin in the urine, which discolours the urine red. The severity of the symptoms varies from one individual to another, and in some cases the combination of symptoms may be life threatening. In severe attacks, there may be breathing difficulties due to the respiratory muscles being affected, and the function of the kidneys can also be affected. In addition, in type 1 there may be enlargement of the liver (hepatomegaly).

Type 2 is the more severe form of the disorder, and can affect infants with onset occurring from birth to 18 months. It appears to affect males more than females, and is more commonly seen in people affected by diabetes or malnutrition. Symptoms may be triggered by long periods without food, and may include low blood sugar levels (hypoglycaemia) and muscle pain (myalgia). In addition, there may be an irregular heartbeat (arrhythmia), and also thickening (hypertrophy) and enlargement (dilation) of the heart, which is known as cardiomyopathy.

This disorder can be diagnosed on the basis of clinical evaluation, enzyme studies and muscle biopsy. Treatment is symptomatic and supportive. Exercise should be taken in moderation, a diet that is low in proteins and high in carbohydrates is recommended, and affected individuals should also avoid foods with a high fat content. Those affected by this disorder need regular supplies of food and drink, as fasting must be avoided completely. Stress should be kept to a minimum, and it is important for these individuals to keep warm enough. Carnitine supplements may be of benefit to some patients.

Reviewed by Professor M Gardiner

Glutaric aciduria type 1

> **Other names for this condition**
> - GA 1
> - Dicarboxylic aminoaciduria
> - Glutaric acidaemia type 1
> - Glutaryl-CoA dehydrogenase deficiency
> - Glutaryl-coenzyme A dehydrogenase deficiency

Glutaric aciduria is a rare metabolic disorder that belongs to a group of conditions known as organic acidaemias, in which the individual is unable to break down certain proteins, and the result is a build-up of chemicals, usually acids, in the body. In glutaric aciduria type 1, there is a deficiency or an absence of the enzyme glutaryl-CoA dehydrogenase, and this leads to a build-up of glutaric acid. It is the accumulation of this acid that causes the symptoms of this condition.

This disorder is genetically inherited from the parents in an autosomal recessive fashion.

Children with this disorder usually appear normal at birth. There may be some non-specific signs of the condition in early infancy, such as an enlarged head circumference (macrocephaly), mildly decreased muscle tone (hypotonia) and irritability. However, because these signs are non-specific, the diagnosis is rarely made at this stage. The disorder usually presents with a severe illness within the first 2 to 3 years of life, usually precipitated by a common childhood infection. Symptoms include impaired brain function and loss of consciousness (encephalopathy), loss of muscle tone (hypotonia), vomiting, and high levels of glutaric acid in the body tissues. Brain damage may occur following the initial episode, and can result in increased muscle tone (dystonia), which may cause children to position themselves in strange positions and to make involuntary slow writhing or jerky movements of the body and limbs. Fits (seizures) may also subsequently occur, along with spasms that cause the head and heels to be bent backwards while the rest of the body is bowed forwards. Acute encephalopathy may recur in acute episodes that are brought on by childhood illnesses associated with fever. Treatment of these episodes should be rapid, as a build-up of glutaric acid can cause further brain damage.

This disorder is diagnosed on the basis of urine and blood tests to detect the presence of glutaric acid and related compounds. The diagnosis can be confirmed by measuring the level of glutaryl-CoA dehydrogenase enzyme activity in the white blood cells, or by obtaining a skin biopsy specimen. Treatment of glutaric aciduria involves carnitine supplementation and careful management of common childhood illnesses that have the potential to cause brain damage. Some centres also use protein-restricted diets. Common childhood illnesses are usually managed by temperature control and the use of high-carbohydrate drinks. If these are not tolerated, intravenous administration of dextrose and carnitine may be necessary. If the disorder is diagnosed and treated before the onset of the initial acute episode, brain damage can be prevented, allowing normal growth and development.

Prenatal diagnosis is possible, and genetic counselling may be of benefit to affected individuals and their families.

Reviewed by Dr A Chakrapani

Isovaleric acidaemia

Other names for this condition
- IVA
- Isovaleric acid CoA dehydrogenase deficiency
- Isovalericacidaemia
- Isovaleryl CoA carboxylase deficiency
- IVD deficiency

Isovaleric acidaemia is a rare metabolic disorder that belongs to a group of conditions known as the organic acidaemias. It is caused by a deficiency of the enzyme isovaleryl CoA dehydrogenase (IVD), which is needed by the body to break down the amino acid leucine. In the body, leucine is then taken from the bloodstream and converted into isovaleryl CoA. If there is a deficiency of the IVD enzyme, isovaleryl CoA accumulates in the blood and is converted into other compounds that are toxic to the body. One of these compounds is an organic acid known as isovaleric acid, which causes a characteristic odour when individuals have an acute metabolic crisis.

This disorder is genetically inherited from the parents in an autosomal recessive fashion.

Isovaleric acidaemia occurs in two forms – an acute and a chronic intermittent form. Symptoms may present at any time between the first week of life and adolescence, and affected individuals may experience vomiting, have a poor appetite and become lethargic. Infants with this disorder may have a low body temperature (hypothermia) and shake or tremble. Those affected by the disorder tend to show an aversion to foods containing protein, and they usually experience acute metabolic crises, which are most commonly triggered by an infection or overconsumption of high-protein foods. These crises are usually followed by severe acidity and the presence of organic compounds known as ketones in the blood and body tissues (ketoacidosis). In some cases, affected individuals may lapse into a coma. These episodes become less frequent as the child gets older. In some cases, if there is a deficiency causing other chemical reactions in the body to be disrupted, ammonia may accumulate in the blood (hyperammonaemia), which can lead to brain damage.

Isovaleric acidaemia is generally diagnosed in the first weeks of life on the basis of a clinical evaluation and a medical family history. Laboratory tests include tests on specific white blood cells (leukocytes) or cultured skin cells (fibroblasts) to confirm deficient enzyme activity, and other tests to reveal symptoms of the disorder such as ketoacidosis and hyperammonaemia. Prenatal diagnosis by amniocentesis or chorionic villus sampling (CVS) is available. At some centres the disorder can be diagnosed by a newborn screening programme using tandem mass spectrometry (TMS).

Treatment of this disorder includes a leucine-restricted diet with L-carnitine supplements. In addition, glycine is administered to allow normal growth and development, and this treatment is also life-saving. Other treatment is symptomatic and supportive. Genetic counselling is recommended for individuals affected by this disorder.

Reviewed by Ms J Gick

Medium-chain acyl CoA dehydrogenase deficiency

Other names for this condition

- MCAD deficiency
- MCADD
- Non-ketotic hypoglycaemia and carnitine deficiency due to MCADD

This disorder belongs to a group of conditions known as fatty acid oxidation disorders, where there is a deficiency of a mitochondrial enzyme. Due to the enzyme deficiency it is difficult for the body to break down fatty acids to produce energy. In MCAD deficiency, the specific mitochondrial enzyme needed to break down medium-chain fatty acids is deficient.

This disorder is genetically inherited from the parents in an autosomal recessive fashion.

Symptoms of this disorder tend to appear between 3 and 15 months, although a few cases have been documented in which a later onset occurred. Symptoms generally occur in unexplained recurrent episodes of stress, commonly known as metabolic crises, generally in response to an infection and/or a period of fasting. Typical symptoms during these metabolic crises include low blood sugar levels (hypoglycaemia), lack of energy (lethargy), and fits (seizures). If the metabolic crisis is severe, the symptoms may include breathing difficulties (respiratory distress) and/or problems with heart function (cardiorespiratory arrest), and possibly unresponsiveness and unconsciousness (coma). These metabolic crises tend to vary from one individual to another with regard to symptoms and severity. Sudden, severe, life-threatening symptoms can occur at any time in undiagnosed individuals, causing coma and/or death if not treated quickly.

In individuals with MCAD deficiency, fatty acids may accumulate in the liver and brain, high levels of ammonia may build up in the blood (hyperammonaemia), the liver may be enlarged (hepatomegaly), and fluid can accumulate around the brain (cerebral oedema). In some children, this disorder can lead to delays in mental and physical development.

Treatment of this disorder aims to prevent and control the acute metabolic crises. Affected individuals are at high risk if there is no intake of food for longer than the recommended time,* so frequent consumption of food is necessary. In addition, L-carnitine supplements have proved to be beneficial for some families, and are commonly given in some countries. Once MCAD deficiency has been diagnosed, the prognosis for individuals is extremely good.

Reviewed by Dr JH Walter

* Current recommendations in the UK:

0–4 months	6 hours
4–8 months	8 hours
8–12 months	10 hours
> 12 months	12 hours

Methylglutaconic aciduria (3) – type 2

Other names for this condition
- Barth syndrome
- Cardioskeletal myopathy with neutropenia and abnormal mitochondria
- Cardioskeletal myopathy, Barth type
- Endocardial fibroelastosis, type 2
- MGA type II
- X-linked cardioskeletal myopathy and neutropenia

Methylglutaconic aciduria (3) type 2 is more commonly known as Barth syndrome. This disorder is caused by changes in a protein called cardiolipin. This is a very important component of the mitochondria, which themselves act as powerhouses for our cells. As a result, the disease affects tissues which are very dependent on energy, such as heart and skeletal muscle, causing 'cardioskeletal myopathy.' Barth syndrome is easily mistaken for other mitochondrial diseases, and is often diagnosed quite late.

This disorder is genetically transmitted by X-linked inheritance.

Symptoms of this condition may become apparent at any time from birth to 10 years of age, but usually appear during infancy or early childhood. The main symptoms include weakening of the heart muscle, which usually leads to enlargement of the lower chambers (dilated cardiomyopathy). There may also be thickening of the heart with overgrowth of fibrous and elastic tissues (endocardial fibroelastosis), or dilation of just part of the heart (left ventricular non-compaction). The dilation and thickening of the heart leads to a reduced ability to pump blood around the body (cardiac failure), and can cause breathlessness and fatigue on exertion, bluish discoloration of the skin (cyanosis) and irregular heartbeats (arrhythmias). Symptoms of heart failure are usually worst during infancy, but may improve and then deteriorate again during puberty. Arrhythmias are particularly common during the teenage years. There may be reduced levels of muscle tone (hypotonia) and muscle weakness, as well as a delay in physical development and growth, with 'failure to thrive' and short stature (although boys continue to grow late, and consequently often end up well grown). Some children may show falls in their blood sugar level (hypoglycaemia). Many children have food cravings, especially for savoury foods such as cheese, pickles and crisps. There are frequently low levels of the white blood cells known as neutrophils, which help to fight infections. This leads to a weakened immune system, and affected individuals become prone to infections and mouth ulcers.

There are increased levels of certain acids in the blood and urine, particularly 3-methylglutaconic acid and 3-methylglutaric acid. There may also be low levels of cholesterol in the blood of affected individuals. Some individuals may have mild learning disabilities. The range and severity of symptoms can vary markedly from one person to another. For example, some children may only rarely have a low neutrophil count.

Treatment of this disorder may include medications to improve the heart condition and prompt antibiotic treatment when infections do occur. For individuals who have frequent infections or mouth ulcers, the drug granulocyte-colony stimulating factor (G-CSF) can be given regularly to stimulate white cell production. Carnitine supplementation is *not* recommended in patients with Barth syndrome. Pantothenic acid has been reported to lead to improvement, but only in a small proportion of patients.

Early diagnosis is important so that the appropriate treatment can be given, otherwise potentially life-threatening complications may develop. Complications can also develop throughout the course of the disease, and may include severe infections and heart failure. If there is serious deterioration of the heart, cardiac transplant may be required.

Reviewed by Dr C Steward

Methylmalonic acidaemia

Other names for this condition

- Methylmalonic aciduria

This disorder belongs to a group of conditions known as organic acid disorders, in which there is a build-up of organic acids in the body. Individuals with an organic acid disorder have a chemical imbalance in their body that can be toxic. Organic acids play an important role in the breakdown of fats, sugars and protein for use by the body or for storage. Methylmalonic acidaemia is caused by a deficiency or absence of an enzyme that is required for the metabolism of certain amino acids, namely isoleucine, valine, threonine and methionine, as well as odd-chain fatty acids.

There are at least seven different forms of methylmalonic acidaemia:

- Mut(0)
- Mut(-)
- CblA
- CblB
- CblC
- CblD
- CblF.

The Cbl disorders result from impaired cobalamin metabolism. CbIA and CbIB are caused by defects in the pathway of adenosylcobalamin synthesis, and are usually responsive to cobalamin supplements.

All of the above forms result in methylmalonic acidaemia with the same symptoms, except for CblC, CblD and CblF, which result in combined methylmalonic acidaemia and homocystinuria. This condition is described in a separate summary (*see* p. 7).

Methylmalonic acidaemia is genetically inherited from the parents in an autosomal recessive fashion.

Survival and neurological outcome in individuals with methylmalonic acidaemia are determined by the response to doses of cobalamin and the age at onset of symptoms. Patients with early onset and non-responsiveness to cobalamin have higher disease severity, a median survival of 6 years, and a poorer neurological and cognitive outcome. Cobalamin-non-responsive patients are at increased risk of developing new neurological symptoms and signs with age. These develop following episodes of acute metabolic decompensation.

The onset of this condition is usually during the first few months of life, although some individuals present with symptoms later in childhood. Symptoms may include lethargy, failure to grow and gain weight (failure to thrive), recurrent vomiting, dehydration, respiratory distress, low muscle tone (hypotonia), delay in mental development, fits (seizures), low blood sugar levels (hypoglycaemia) and an enlarged liver (hepatomegaly). There will be a build-up of acids in the body (metabolic acidosis), with abnormally high levels of methylmalonic acid in the blood and urine. There are sometimes high levels of the amino acid glycine in the blood and urine (hyperglycinaemia and hyperglycinuria), and also of ketones in the blood and urine (ketonaemia and ketonuria), as well as of ammonia in the blood (hyperammonaemia). There may also be reduced numbers of platelets (thrombocytopenia) and white blood cells (neutropenia) in the blood. Acute episodes may include drowsiness and seizures, with subsequent developmental delays. If treatment is not undertaken, coma and death may occur.

Future acute attacks of metabolic acidosis or the exacerbation of symptoms may be caused by illnesses such as infections, or by the consumption of large amounts of protein.

Individuals with this disorder should alert their physician to the possibility of stroke if they have abnormal tonicity of muscle, characterised by prolonged, repetitive muscle contractions that may cause twisting or jerking movements, difficulty in swallowing, and speech difficulties. They should also alert him or her if a condition is present that is marked by abnormal movements of the body that include combined jerky movements, especially of the arms, legs and face, loss of coordination, and slow, writhing, involuntary movements of flexion, extension, rotation of the fingers and hands, and sometimes of the toes and feet.

Prenatal diagnosis is available by amniocentesis, in which a sample of the fluid surrounding the fetus is withdrawn and analysed. Alternatively, chorionic villus sampling (CVS) is available, in which a portion of the placenta is removed and examined. The disorder can be identified at birth by the newborn screening programmes available in some countries. Many infants are diagnosed during the first few weeks of life, using a thorough clinical evaluation, a detailed family history and a variety of specialised tests.

Long-term treatment consists of a low-protein diet that must be followed carefully in order to limit intake of the amino acids, and the avoidance of fasting. Cobalamin, carnitine and vitamin B_{12} supplements are sometimes given, as there can be an associated secondary deficiency, and they can also aid the metabolism of some fatty acids and amino acids. Other treatment may be symptomatic and supportive.

Treatment of an acute episode should restrict any further intake of protein in order to prevent any additional increase in acid levels. Intravenous fluids and bicarbonate should be given to help to reduce the acid levels in the body. Dialysis may be needed if the acid levels are extremely high. Glucose and other nutritional supplements are usually given to prevent the breakdown of any stored isoleucine, valine, threonine and methionine that would increase the acid levels further. Sometimes vitamin B_{12} and carnitine are given, as they play a role in the metabolism of certain fatty acids and proteins.

Reviewed by Dr JH Walter

Multiple acyl CoA dehydrogenase deficiency

> **Other names for this condition**
> - Deficiency of electron transfer flavoprotein
> - Deficiency of electron transfer flavoprotein–ubiquinone oxidoreductase
> - GA II
> - Glutaric acidaemia II
> - Glutaric aciduria II
> - MADD
> - Multiple acyl CoA dehydrogenation deficiency

Multiple acyl CoA dehydrogenase deficiency is a rare disorder that belongs to a group of conditions known as the organic acidaemias. It can be caused by a deficiency in either the electron transfer flavoprotein (ETF) enzyme or the ETF–ubiquinone oxidoreductase (ETF–QO) enzyme. This results in the accumulation of organic acids in the blood and urine. There are two forms of multiple acyl CoA dehydrogenase deficiency:

- a neonatal form in which the enzyme is completely absent, and that is often fatal during the newborn period
- a late-onset form which is less severe and that can present at any age.

This disorder is genetically inherited from the parents in an autosomal recessive fashion.

Symptoms of the neonatal form of this disorder include extremely low blood sugar levels (severe hypoglycaemia), low muscle tone (hypotonia) and respiratory distress (where the respiratory system is in danger of not being able to keep up with the requirements for oxygen and gas exchange). Individuals affected by this disorder may have characteristic facial features, including an enlarged head, ear abnormalities, a high forehead and a flat nasal bridge. Other symptoms include an enlarged liver (hepatomegaly), kidney abnormalities, genital abnormalities and a distinctive odour. The symptoms of the late-onset form vary widely, and may include low blood sugar levels (hypoglycaemia) and periods of nausea, vomiting and weakness.

Multiple acyl CoA dehydrogenase deficiency can be diagnosed by urine analysis to test for the organic acids glutaric acid, ethylmalonic acid, adipic acid and isovaleric acid. A skin biopsy can be used to confirm the diagnosis by demonstrating abnormal enzyme activity in cultured fibroblast cells. This disorder can also be diagnosed by newborn screening programmes available in certain countries. Prenatal diagnosis may be possible by measuring the glutaric acid levels in the amniotic fluid, and by enzyme analysis with chorionic villus sampling (CVS).

This disorder is usually treated with a high-carbohydrate, low-protein diet that is also low in fat. In addition, riboflavin, glycine and carnitine supplements may be prescribed. Affected individuals should eat regularly, and may need to consume food during the night to avoid low blood sugar levels. Early diagnosis and treatment may change the natural history of this disorder.

Reviewed by Dr JH Walter

Propionic acidaemia

Other names for this condition

- Hyperglycinaemia with ketoacidosis and lactic acidosis, propionic type
- Ketotic glycinaemia
- PCC deficiency
- Propionyl CoA carboxylase deficiency

Propionic acidaemia is an organic acid disorder that is caused by deficiency of an enzyme known as propionyl CoA carboxylase (PCC). This enzyme is involved in the breakdown of the amino acids isoleucine, valine, threonine and methionine, and it has two subunits, α and β.

This disorder is genetically inherited from the parents in an autosomal recessive fashion.

Propionic acidaemia usually presents in the first few weeks of life. However, in some cases the disorder may only become apparent in infancy or later. It is believed that breastfeeding may be associated with a later onset. Symptoms include low muscle tone (hypotonia), lethargy, feeding difficulties, vomiting, and failure to grow or gain weight (failure to thrive). Other symptoms may include seizures, and other findings may include abnormally high levels of acid (acidosis) and increased levels of the amino acid glycine in the blood and urine (hyperglycinaemia and hyper-glycinuria). There may also be an accumulation of ketone bodies in the tissues and fluids (ketosis), and high levels of ammonia in the blood (hyperammonaemia). Other findings may include low levels of circulating platelets (thrombocytopenia) and of certain white blood cells known as neutrophils (neutropenia). Symptoms may be worsened by infections, constipation or overconsumption of high-protein foods. Without appropriate treatment, these symptoms can progress to coma and other life-threatening complications.

Propionic acidaemia is usually diagnosed on the basis of a clinical evaluation, routine laboratory tests and specialised tests to demonstrate the deficient activity of the propionyl CoA carboxylase enzyme. Prenatal diagnosis is possible by testing the amniotic fluid for abnormal enzyme activity or by analysing a portion of the placenta by chorionic villus sampling (CVS). In some instances this disorder can be diagnosed at birth through newborn screening programmes.

Early diagnosis and treatment should help to reduce complications, but affected children may still have problems, including pancreatitis, cardiomyopathy, neurolo-gical problems (including slow development) and recurrent episodes of acute illness.

Treatment consists of a low-protein diet, which may be supplemented with artificial proteins. In some cases carnitine may need to be supplemented with L-carnitine. If the disorder is severe, the patient may require dialysis to remove waste products from the blood. If an acute episode occurs, treatment may include fluid and electrolyte therapy, and antibiotics to prevent or treat infections. Other treatments may include the administration of biotin, as well as various services, including special education and occupational therapy. All other treatment aims to provide relief of any symptoms and support in the care of the affected individual. All families should be offered genetic counselling.

Reviewed by Professor J Leonard

Trimethylaminuria syndrome

Other names for this condition
- Fish odour syndrome
- Flavin-containing monooxygenase 2
- 2 FMO adult liver form
- FMO2
- Stale fish syndrome

This disorder is characterised by the inability of the body to break down trimethylamine, which is normally formed in the intestines by bacterial action on certain substances, namely choline (a vitamin B complex) and trimethylamine oxide. Trimethylamine is produced in the intestines, and is then transported to the liver and converted into trimethylamine oxide (which has no odour) by the enzyme trimethylamine oxidase. In this disorder, the inability to convert trimethylamine causes an accumulation of the substance in the body, which produces a fishy odour when it is excreted in the urine, sweat and breath.

This disorder is genetically inherited by autosomal dominant inheritance.

The use of L-carnitine in carnitine deficiency syndromes can lead to the symptoms of fish odour syndrome. In addition, athletes sometimes use L-carnitine in the belief that it will enhance their physical strength, and this can also lead to symptoms.

The main symptom of this disorder is a fishy odour when trimethylamine is present at a high concentration, and a more general rotten odour when it is present in low concentrations. The odour is especially prominent in sweat from the armpits and the feet, on the breath and from the urine. Symptoms can occur at any age, and are dependent on the ingestion of specific foods. Sources of choline that can be found in the diet include liver, kidneys, wheatgerm, brewer's yeast, egg yolk and legumes, including broccoli, peas and peanuts. Sources of trimethylamine oxide that can be found in the diet include some species of saltwater fish. The production of trimethylamine may increase around the time of puberty, and also at times of stress and during exercise. In women, trimethylamine production can increase just before or during menstruation, after taking oral contraceptives and around the time of the menopause.

Due to the fact that the main symptom of this condition is production of an odour, there is a possibility that there will be associated psychological and social problems such as depression, social withdrawal, low self-esteem and social exclusion.

In most cases, the odour can be reduced by excluding from the affected individual's diet any foods that contain choline and trimethylamine oxide, giving low doses of antibiotics to reduce the quantity of bacteria in the gut, and using soap with a moderate pH (between 5.5 and 6.5). In addition, a low-protein diet has been found to be of benefit if symptoms do persist. Behavioural counselling is recommended to aid depression and other neurological symptoms, and genetic counselling may also be of benefit. Drugs that interfere with hepatic metabolism should be avoided.

In cases where symptoms are brought on by the use of L-carnitine, a reduction in the dosage can make the odour disappear.

Reviewed by Dr RE Pugh

Chapter 3

Mitochondrial and peroxisomal disorders

Mitochondrial disorders

Mitochondria are small structures that are found in all cells except red blood cells. They contain their own DNA (known as mitochondrial DNA or mtDNA), and are responsible for producing the energy that is needed by the cell to carry out its functions. Any defect in the mitochondria will mean that there is a reduction in the amount of energy produced. This can lead to damage to the cell and ultimately to cell destruction. If this happens throughout the cells of the body, it will lead to failure of the body's systems and cause the symptoms of a mitochondrial disorder. Defects in the genes of the mtDNA are maternally inherited.

Peroxisomal disorders

Peroxisomes are small membrane-bound intracellular organelles containing enzymes that serve many important functions in the body, including β-oxidation of very-long-chain fatty acids (VLCFA), β-oxidation of phytanic acids and β-oxidation of di- and trihydroxycholestanoic acids to chenodeoxycholic acid and cholic acid, which are bile acid precursors. Peroxisomal disorders are classified into two main groups:

1   multiple enzyme deficiencies resulting from disorders of peroxisomal biogenesis
2   single peroxisomal enzyme deficiencies.

Patients who have a disorder of peroxisomal biogenesis lack normal peroxisomes. Four conditions are recognised:

- Zellweger syndrome (ZS)
- neonatal adrenoleukodystrophy (NALD)
- infantile Refsum disease (IRD)
- rhizomelic chondrodysplasia punctata (RCDP).

They are all associated with severely impaired peroxisomal assembly, loss of multiple enzyme activities and multi-system involvement.

Adrenoleukodystrophy – X-linked

Other names for this condition

- Addison–Schilder disease
- Addison disease with cerebral sclerosis
- ALD
- Bronze Schilder's disease
- Encephalitis periaxialis diffusa
- Flatau–Schilder disease
- Melanodermic leukodystrophy
- Myelinoclastic diffuse sclerosis
- Schilder disease
- Schilder encephalitis
- Siewerling–Creutzfeldt disease
- Sudanophilic leukodystrophy (ADL)
- X-ALD

This is an inherited disorder that is characterised by the breakdown or loss of the myelin sheath surrounding the nerve cells in the brain and spinal cord, accompanied by progressive dysfunction of the adrenal gland. This is due to deficiency of a protein known as ABCD1, whose function is still not well understood. One consequence of this defect is a build-up of very-long-chain fatty acids (VLCFAs) in the blood and tissues of the body.

This disorder is genetically inherited by X-linked inheritance.

Female carriers commonly do not show any symptoms, although they may develop much milder symptoms than affected boys later in adult life. Most boys and men affected by the disease will develop adrenal gland failure (Addison's disease) at some stage. In the early stages this often presents with severe vomiting, leading quickly to dehydration, and accompanied by low serum sodium levels. This pattern then tends to be repeated even after minor infections. There may be bronzing of the skin. This needs to be recognised promptly and treated with steroid supplements (hydrocortisone with or without fludrocortisone). Careful neurological follow-up is imperative in boys who have presented with adrenal problems alone.

Some males will never develop any symptoms apart from adrenal problems. However, approximately 90% will later develop one of the neurological forms of ALD. In descending order of frequency, these are as follows:

- childhood cerebral ALD (30–40% of cases)
- adrenomyeloneuropathy (AMN)
- adolescent cerebral ALD.

The first symptoms of childhood cerebral ALD usually appear between the ages of 4 and 10 years, and can include changes in behaviour, such as poor memory, poor performance at school, and loss of emotional control. These symptoms may resemble those of attention deficit hyperactivity disorder (ADHD). Other problems include squints or visual loss, dysarthria (poorly articulated speech), hearing problems, walking difficulties (due to progressive gait and stiffness of the legs), seizures and progressive dementia. Once apparent, this disease often progresses to a severe form within 2 years, and to death within 10 years. Adolescent boys who develop cerebral ALD often show similar symptoms but progress less rapidly.

Adrenomyeloneuropathy (AMN) is a milder adult-onset form that tends to primarily affect the spinal nerves. It typically begins in the third or fourth decades of life. Symptoms may include leg stiffness, progressive spastic paraparesis (stiffness, weakness and/or paralysis) of the lower limbs and ataxia (unsteadiness). Although it is more slowly progressive than the childhood form, AMN can also result in deterioration of brain function.

ALD is diagnosed by a blood test to measure the VLCFAs, although this test is not completely reliable. Very occasionally males with proven ALD may have normal blood levels of VLCFAs. Carrier females may have raised or normal levels of VLCFAs (these tend to decrease with age), and genetic testing is the only way to exclude carrier status when VLCFA levels are normal in women.

Boys who have been shown to have ALD on blood testing but who have no neurological problems are strongly recommended to go on a low-fat diet and to take Lorenzo's oil (which greatly reduces or normalises VLCFA levels), as this may delay progression of the disease. The role of Lorenzo's oil is also being investigated in men with AMN and in symptomatic female carriers. Boys without neurological symptoms are followed up by careful brain scanning (MRI and MRS scans), as bone-marrow transplantation from healthy donors can prevent progression of the disease if performed at an early stage of deterioration. For boys with symptomatic neurological disease, treatment of the neurological symptoms is usually supportive and symptomatic. Genetic counselling is recommended for individuals affected by this disorder.

Reviewed by Dr C Steward

Alper's disease

Other names for this condition

- Alper's diffuse degeneration of cerebral grey matter with hepatic cirrhosis
- Alper's–Huttenlocher syndrome
- Alper's progressive infantile poliodystrophy
- Alper's progressive sclerosing poliodystrophy
- Alper's syndrome
- Christensen's disease
- Christensen–Krabbe disease
- Diffuse cerebral degeneration in infancy
- PNDC
- Poliodystrophia cerebri progressiva
- Progressive cerebral poliodystrophy
- Progressive infantile poliodystrophy
- Progressive neuronal degeneration of childhood with liver disease

---

Alper's disease is a progressive neurological disorder that is believed to be caused by a biochemical defect that leads to cell damage and cell loss in the grey matter of the brain. This damage hinders the transmission of nerve signals both within the brain and from the brain to other parts of the body. A very rare form of Alper's disease occurs in older children and teenagers. Juvenile Alper's disease has a longer time course.

This disorder is inherited in an autosomal recessive fashion. However, it is likely that in some cases different patterns of inheritance may occur. Many affected individuals have an underlying mitochondrial disorder, and recent evidence shows that a number of patients have defects in the *POLG1* gene.

Alper's disease generally presents in early childhood. Symptoms may include a delay in physical and mental development, and infants may not reach developmental milestones such as walking until later than expected. Affected individuals may show a progressive loss of intellectual ability (dementia), and usually suffer from fits (seizures) and muscle jerks. Some individuals may experience hearing difficulties or become deaf. Other signs include a low muscle tone (hypotonia), increased muscle tension leading to exaggerated reflexes, stiffness of the limbs (spasticity), and in some cases paralysis of all four limbs (quadriplegia). In some individuals there may be degeneration of the optic nerve (optic atrophy), which can lead to blindness. Liver problems usually develop later and present with jaundice (yellow discoloration of the skin). Unfortunately, liver disease usually progresses to liver failure. In rare cases, liver disease may be the first sign of the disease. Liver failure and seizures are the main cause of death in Alper's disease. Individuals with this disorder do not usually survive beyond the first decade of life.

There is no single diagnostic test for Alper's disease. The diagnosis is usually made using a combination of a detailed family history, clinical evaluation and a range of specialised tests. In fatal cases, a post-mortem examination of the brain may be the best way to confirm the diagnosis. Alper's disease may be misdiagnosed as liver failure or childhood jaundice.

Unfortunately, liver transplantation is not successful in individuals with this disorder. The aim of treatment is to provide relief of any symptoms and to give support. Stress should be avoided, as it is believed that it can intensify symptoms. Anticonvulsant drugs may be given to help to prevent or control seizures. Sodium valproate should never be given to patients with this disorder, as it may precipitate liver failure. Other medications may be given to relieve pain and to treat infections as appropriate. Physiotherapy may help to increase muscle tone and/or relieve any muscle contractions. Advice may be given on exercise and positioning. Research into the use of L-carnitine and coenzyme Q_{10} as possible treatments is ongoing.

Reviewed by Dr P McKiernan and Dr A Morris

Fumarase deficiency

Other names for this condition
- Fumaric aciduria
- Fumarate hydratase deficiency

Fumarase deficiency is a rare disorder of the Kreb's cycle (also known as the citric acid cycle), a metabolic pathway that is central to the breakdown of carbohydrates, fats and proteins to carbon dioxide and water in order to generate energy. Individuals affected by this disorder develop postnatal neurological problems. Patients who have a more severe form of fumarase deficiency usually develop respiratory difficulties, and this results in their life expectancy not extending beyond early childhood, whereas patients who are less severely affected develop non-progressive brain problems and survive into adolescence or adulthood.

This disorder is genetically inherited from the parents in an autosomal recessive fashion.

The symptoms of fumarase deficiency vary depending on the severity of the case. Infants sometimes suffer from mild lactic acidosis and mild hyperammonaemia, although older children are not generally affected in this way. General symptoms include an unusually small head (microcephaly), sight problems, poor feeding, weight loss, poor muscle tension (hypotonia) and an inability to hold the head up. In some cases, an unborn child may develop water on the brain (hydrocephalus), or the transverse fibres that link the two cerebral hemispheres of the brain may be partly or completely missing (agenesis of the corpus callosum). This is sometimes associated with an excessive amount of fluid surrounding the fetus from approximately week 20 of pregnancy. Children born with this condition may have low-set ears and a small jawbone, and a CT scan may reveal a 'smooth brain' (lissencephaly), a condition in which the brain develops with no outer grooves, large ventricles, and is generally smaller than usual. Prenatal diagnosis is available.

Treatment depends on the severity of the condition and is mainly supportive. It may be beneficial for the individual to be placed on a dialysis machine which can be used to remove certain amino acids that are precursors of fumarate.

Reviewed by Dr G Besley

Kearns–Sayre syndrome

Other names for this condition

- CPEO with myopathy
- CPEO with ragged red fibres
- Chronic progressive external ophthalmoplegia and myopathy
- Chronic progressive external ophthalmoplegia with ragged red fibres
- Kearns–Sayre disease
- KSS
- Mitochondrial cytopathy, Kearns–Sayre type
- Oculocraniosomatic neuromuscular disease
- Oculocraniosomatic syndrome (obsolete)
- Ophthalmoplegia plus syndrome
- Ophthalmoplegia, pigmentary degeneration of the retina and cardiomyopathy

Kearns–Sayre syndrome is a rare neuromuscuclar disorder that belongs to a group of rare disorders known as the mitochondrial encephalomyopathies. These disorders are characterised by a defect in the genetic material of the mitochondria (the cell structures that release energy), which impairs the functioning of the muscles and the brain. In many cases, tests reveal a deletion involving the mitochondrial DNA. In some cases Kearns–Sayre syndrome may be associated with other disorders or conditions.

This disorder is most often caused by a deletion in the mitochondrial DNA, and sometimes a duplication is found. It is most often a sporadic event, but occasionally may be inherited from the maternal line (when there is a fault in the mitochondrial DNA).

Kearns–Sayre syndrome typically shows onset of features before the age of 20 years. The eyes are often affected, with paralysis of the eye muscles (chronic progressive external ophthalmoplegia) and an accumulation of abnormal pigment at the back of the eye (pigmentary retinopathy). Another characteristic feature is abnormal heartbeat rhythm (due to cardiac conduction defects). Neurologically, affected individuals have poor balance and may have muscle weakness. As with other mitochondrial disorders, in Kearns–Sayre syndrome many other body systems may be affected to a variable extent, leading to short stature, an underactive parathyroid gland, ovarian or testicular failure and hearing loss. There may be progressive loss of intellectual skills similar to that in dementia.

Kearns–Sayre syndrome is diagnosed on the basis of a clinical evaluation and specialised tests. There are no specific treatments, but monitoring of the multi-system effects allows appropriate symptomatic treatments.

Reviewed by Dr M Cleary

Leigh syndrome

Other names for this condition
- Leigh disease
- Necrotising encephalomyelopathy (of Leigh)
- Subacute necrotising encephalomyelopathy
- SNE

Patients with Leigh syndrome usually develop symptoms in the first few months of life, although in some cases onset of symptoms may not occur until later in childhood or even (occasionally) in adulthood. Affected individuals characteristically suffer degeneration of the nervous system as a result of impaired energy production by the mitochondria of brain cells. Mitochondria are the cell's 'batteries', and they produce energy in the form of ATP (adenosine triphosphate), mainly through the enzymatic processes of oxidative phosphorylation (OXPHOS).

The enzyme defect is genetically inherited from the parents in one of a number of different ways, depending on the precise genetic defect in the individual. It is thought that most cases of Leigh syndrome are genetically inherited from the parents in an autosomal recessive manner.

Approximately 20% of cases of Leigh syndrome are caused by defects in genes located within the mitochondria. These genes are collectively known as the mitochondrial genome or mitochondrial DNA (mtDNA). The mtDNA is only passed down from mothers to their children, because mtDNA from the sperm is not passed on to the fertilised egg. Defects in mtDNA are therefore described as being maternally inherited. This means that girls will always pass on a defect in the mtDNA to their children, whereas boys will never pass on such a defect.

The final way in which Leigh syndrome may be passed on genetically is by X-linked inheritance. This applies to some cases of pyruvate dehydrogenase (PDH) deficiency.

In the classical form of Leigh syndrome, symptoms usually appear before the age of 2 years. The initial symptoms may include a loss of previously acquired skills such as head control and the ability to suck. There may also be a loss of appetite, vomiting, general irritability and abnormal crying. If the onset is later in childhood, the symptoms that may occur include difficulty in articulating words, a loss of intellectual skills and difficulty coordinating movements (ataxia). As the disease progresses, further symptoms may include generalised weakness, lack of muscle tone (hypotonia), clumsiness and tremors. Affected individuals may develop problems with breathing and sometimes with swallowing. Visual problems that may occur include rapid eye movement (nystagmus), crossed eyes (strabismus) and degeneration of the optic nerve (optic atrophy). Further neurological development is delayed. Other organs that may be affected are the heart (hypertrophic cardiomyopathy, in which the heart is abnormally enlarged) and the kidneys.

In the adult form of Leigh syndrome, symptoms usually begin during adolescence or adulthood with disturbances to the vision, such as blurring, colour blindness and/ or progressive loss of vision, due to degeneration of the optic nerve (optic atrophy).

Later, in midlife, other symptoms may appear, including difficulty in coordinating movements (ataxia), muscle spasm, seizures and dementia.

The underlying cause of Leigh syndrome is an inherited defect of energy production. Affected individuals may have a biochemical defect in one or more of the OXPHOS enzyme complexes (complex I, II, III, IV or V) or in the PDH enzyme. Tests that may be used to confirm the diagnosis include measurement of lactate levels in blood and cerebrospinal fluid (CSF), magnetic resonance imaging (MRI) of the brain, and muscle and skin biopsies to measure the activities of the OXPHOS and PDH enzymes.

Unfortunately, there is no curative treatment for Leigh syndrome. Some doctors may try one of a number of vitamin cofactors (such as biotin, thiamine, riboflavin and coenzyme Q_{10}), because very occasionally a patient improves with vitamin therapy. If there are high levels of lactate in the blood, sodium bicarbonate may be helpful. This may need to be given intravenously in the acute setting, but is sometimes given by mouth if the patient has persistent lactic acidosis. Individuals with a deficiency of the PDH enzyme may be recommended to switch to a high-fat, low-carbohydrate (ketogenic) diet. Other treatment aims are supportive, to provide relief from distressing symptoms. For example, drugs may be needed to control seizures or muscle spasms or to reduce nausea and vomiting.

The prognosis is extremely variable and does not appear to be closely correlated with the underlying biochemical or genetic defect. There tends to be a stepwise decline in function over the years, with periods of plateauing or even improvement followed by periods of loss of skills. Loss of skills may follow intercurrent infections, or be triggered by some general anaesthetics, so children with Leigh syndrome should only be anaesthetised in a specialist centre by anaesthetists who are experienced in the management of patients with mitochondrial disorders. For some patients (particularly those with early onset) there may be rapid progression of disease leading to death within a few years of diagnosis, whereas other patients may survive into adulthood. It is difficult to predict the likely pattern of disease progression in individual cases at the time of diagnosis, although this may become clearer in the ensuing months. Progression of the adult form tends to be much slower than that of the classical form, which begins in infancy.

Several research groups in the UK and around the world are actively trying to find cures for Leigh syndrome and other mitochondrial disorders.

Reviewed by Dr S Rahman

Mitochondrial encephalopathy, lactic acidosis and stroke-like episodes

Other names for this condition
- MELAS
- Mitochondrial myopathy, encephalopathy, lactic acidosis and stroke-like episodes
- Myopathy, mitochondrial encephalopathy – lactic acidosis – stroke

Mitochondrial encephalopathy, lactic acidosis and stroke-like episodes are more commonly referred to as MELAS. This disorder is a form of dementia and belongs to a group of conditions known as mitochondrial disorders. Mitochondria are small structures that are found in all cells except red blood cells, and are responsible for producing energy to enable the cell to function. The mitochondria break down sugars, fatty acids and carbohydrates in order to release energy. If there is a defect in the functioning of the mitochondria, this will lead to a reduction in the amount of energy that is produced. In MELAS, a defect in the mitochondria causes brain dysfunction (encephalopathy), seizures, dementia, muscle disease, a build-up of lactic acid in the blood (lactic acidosis) and temporary local paralysis (stroke-like episodes).

MELAS is thought to be genetically inherited by a method known as maternal mitochondrial inheritance. However, in some cases the condition has occurred for no known reason (in which case it is described as spontaneous).

The symptoms of this disorder can appear at any time from birth to adolescence, although some individuals develop symptoms later, in adulthood. The severity of the symptoms depends on the number of mitochondria per cell that carry the mutation, and this figure is variable. Symptoms commonly include the occurrence of stroke-like episodes, which begin with vomiting, headaches and seizures. As the episodes progress there may also be a loss of function on one side of the body (hemiplegia), visual disturbances, and difficulties in speaking or understanding others (aphasia). These episodes may be followed by a temporary loss of function and/or loss of vision on one side, for a period of time ranging from several hours to several weeks. In addition to the stroke-like episodes, there is commonly a build-up of lactic acid in the blood (lactic acidosis), muscle weakness, a lack of muscle tone (hypotonia) and a progressive loss of intellectual and mental capabilities (dementia). This disorder may affect the eye, abnormalities of which include damage to cells in the eye due to the overproduction of pigmentation (retinitis pigmentosa), paralysis of the eye muscles (ophthalmoplegia) and degeneration of the optic nerve (optic atrophy), droopy eyelids (ptosis) and severe visual loss. Other symptoms may include a short stature, insensitivity to pain, progressive loss of hearing due to dysfunction of the inner ear (sensorineural deafness/nerve deafness), speech defects, heart abnormalities (cardiomyopathy) and dilation of the ventricles in the brain.

MELAS can be diagnosed on the basis of blood tests, urine tests, cultured skin fibroblast assays and muscle biopsies to detect the genetic defect. The aims of treatment for this condition are to provide relief of symptoms and supportive care. Anticonvulsant medication may be given to control and help to prevent seizures. Physiotherapy may also be of benefit in relieving muscle stiffness and weakness. Sensorineural deafness has been successfully treated with a cochlear implant. Coenzyme Q_{10}, riboflavin and carnitine are sometimes given, as they may possibly help to improve general mitochondrial function.

Reviewed by Dr G Besley

Mitochondrial respiratory chain complex IV

Other names for this condition
- Complex IV deficiency
- COX deficiency
- Cytochrome C oxidase deficiency
- Deficiency of mitochondrial respiratory chain complex IV

Mitochondrial respiratory chain complex IV is a rare disorder characterised by a deficiency of an important enzyme known as cytochrome C oxidase (COX), which is found in mitochondria. COX is a complex protein that consists of subunits controlled by both nuclear and mitochondrial genes. Mitochondria are small structures within cells that are responsible for producing energy to enable the cells to function. In some cases the COX deficiency may be limited to the skeletal muscle tissues, or to the organ and/or connective tissues, while in other cases the deficiency may be generalised.

There are four forms of this disorder:

- COX deficiency, benign infantile mitochondrial myopathy type
- COX deficiency, French-Canadian type
- COX deficiency, infantile mitochondrial myopathy type
- Leigh disease (*see* p. 44 for a summary).

This disorder may be inherited from the nuclear genes of the parents in an autosomal recessive fashion. In some cases the disorder may result from abnormal mitochondrial genes. This is a more complex situation in terms of patterns of inheritance.

Symptoms of COX deficiency vary from one case to another. COX deficiency of the benign infantile mitochondrial myopathy type is caused by a deficiency of cytochrome C oxidase that may be limited to the skeletal muscle tissues. The heart and kidneys are not affected. Affected individuals may experience lactic acidosis episodes, when levels of lactic acid in the blood become abnormally high. If this condition is left untreated, it is possible that life-threatening complications will occur. However, within the first few years of life, with appropriate treatment, affected individuals may recover from this form of the disorder.

COX deficiency of the infantile mitochondrial myopathy type is caused by a deficiency of cytochrome C oxidase that affects the skeletal muscle tissues as well as several other tissues, such as the organs and/or connective tissues. Symptoms generally begin within the first few weeks of life, and may include muscle weakness, heart problems (cardiomyopathy) and kidney abnormalities. In some cases, individuals fail to gain weight (failure to thrive), have poor muscle tone (hypotonia), exhibit a weak cry and experience difficulties in sucking, swallowing and/or breathing. Other symptoms include episodes of lactic acidosis, which can lead to respiratory difficulties and kidney dysfunction. De Toni–Fanconi–Debré syndrome, a condition that causes kidney abnormalities, may also be present. Symptoms due to De Toni–Fanconi–Debré syndrome may include excessive thirst (polydipsia), excessive urination (polyuria), and excessive excretion of glucose, phosphates, amino acids, bicarbonate, calcium and water in the urine.

COX deficiency of the French-Canadian type affects skeletal muscle tissues, connective tissue and brain tissue. Affected individuals may demonstrate developmental delay, low muscle tone (hypotonia), some characteristic facial features, Leigh's disease, crossing of the eyes (strabismus), impaired ability to control voluntary movements (ataxia), accumulation of fats within the liver and degeneration of the liver (microvesicular steatosis). In some cases there may be episodes of lactic acidosis, which can lead to life-threatening complications.

Leigh disease is a generalised form of COX deficiency that is characterised by progressive degeneration of the brain and abnormalities of other organs of the body. (For a summary of this disorder, *see* p. 44.)

Diagnosis is made postnatally on the basis of a clinical evaluation, characteristic findings and a range of specialised tests. Treatment of mitochondrial respiratory chain complex IV aims to provide relief of any symptoms and support in the care of the individual. Treatment options may need to be planned by a wide range of specialists. In COX deficiency of the benign infantile mitochondrial myopathy type, early diagnosis and prompt intensive treatment that is maintained until the individual has recovered from the disorder are important.

Reviewed by Dr G Besley

Pearson's syndrome

Other names for this condition
- Pearson marrow–pancreas syndrome
- Sideroblastic anaemia with marrow-cell vacuolisation and exocrine pancreatic dysfunction

This disorder belongs to a group of conditions known as mitochondrial disorders. Mitochondria are small structures within cells that are responsible for producing energy to enable the cells to function. They break down sugars, fatty acids and carbohydrates in order to release energy. If there is a defect in the functioning of the mitochondria, this will lead to a reduction in the amount of energy that is produced. This can lead to cells being unable to perform their function, causing the symptoms of a mitochondrial disorder. Pearson's syndrome mainly affects the pancreas and the bone marrow, which produces blood cells.

This disorder is genetically transmitted by maternal mitochondrial inheritance.

Symptoms of Pearson's syndrome commonly appear during the first year of life, although some individuals have been diagnosed as late as 7 years of age. Symptoms may include failure to grow and gain weight (failure to thrive), a pallid appearance, muscle weakness (myopathy), vomiting, lethargy, an enlarged liver (hepatomegaly) and difficulty in coordinating muscle movements (ataxia). Blood tests usually show that there are low levels of white blood cells (neutropenia), red blood cells (anaemia) and platelets (thrombocytopenia). Affected individuals may develop what is known as aplastic anaemia when the levels of all three types of blood cells (red cells, white cells and platelets) are abnormally low. There are problems with the functioning of the pancreas that can result in malabsorption of food and chronic diarrhoea. There may also be a build-up of acids in the body (metabolic acidosis), especially lactic acid, and there can be problems with the functioning of the liver and the kidneys.

It is vital to distinguish Pearson's syndrome from aplastic anaemia, as bone-marrow transplantation is contraindicated in Pearson's syndrome but is often curative in aplastic anaemia.

Clinical diagnosis is based on the demonstration of ring sideroblasts in a bone-marrow examination. Many bone-marrow cells also have vacuoles within them. Treatment for affected individuals aims to provide relief of any symptoms and support in the care of the individual. The anaemia often requires repeated blood transfusions. Both anaemia and pancreatic function may improve with age. If there are high levels of acid in the body, fluids and bicarbonate should be given in order to reduce them.

Individuals with this disorder rarely reach school age, due to complications such as infections, persistent high levels of acid in the body or liver failure. Those who do recover from the anaemia tend to go on to develop Kearns–Sayre syndrome (*see* p. 43).

Reviewed by Dr C Steward

Pyruvate dehydrogenase deficiency

Other names for this condition

- Alaninuria
- Congenital infantile lactic acidosis
- Intermittent ataxia with lactic acidosis
- Intermittent ataxia with pyruvate dehydrogenase deficiency
- Lactic and pyruvate acidaemia with carbohydrate sensitivity
- Lactic and pyruvate acidaemia with episodic ataxia and weakness
- PDCD
- PDD deficiency
- PDH deficiency
- Pyruvate dehydrogenase complex deficiency

This is a disorder of carbohydrate metabolism (the breakdown of sugars, including glucose). In this condition there is an absence or a deficiency of the pyruvate dehydrogenase complex, so the breakdown of pyruvate to form acetyl CoA is impaired. The pyruvate dehydrogenase complex consists of three separate enzymes:

- E1 – pyruvate decarboxylase
- E2 – dihydrolipoyl transacetylase
- E3 – dihydrolipoyl dehydrogenase.

There may be a deficiency of any one of these separate enzymes, which in turn leads to a deficiency of the pyruvate dehydrogenase complex. The most commonly occurring single deficiency that causes pyruvate dehydrogenase deficiency is E1 deficiency. Around 25% of individuals with a condition known as Leigh disease show defects in the pyruvate dehydrogenase complex.

In general, pyruvate dehydrogenase deficiency is genetically inherited by X-linked inheritance. A few cases of this disorder have been found to be inherited in an autosomal recessive fashion, and the disorder has also been reported to occur sporadically for no known reason.

The range and severity of symptoms in this condition vary widely, due to the fact that there may be anything from a complete absence of enzyme activity to between 2% and 40% of the normal enzyme activity levels. This means that some individuals present with severe acidosis in the first few days after birth, some with chronic moderate lactic acidaemia, and some with recurrent episodes of muscle incoordination (ataxia).

Symptoms may include a build-up of acids in the body (metabolic acidosis), with abnormally high levels of lactic acid, although these may only be seen during acute episodes. The cerebrospinal fluid surrounding the brain and spinal cord also contains raised levels of lactic acid (lactic acidosis). Sometimes there are high levels of ammonia in the blood (hyperammonaemia) and raised levels of organic acids, lactic acid and pyruvate in the urine. In addition, there may be a loss of muscle tone (hypotonia), a delay in physical and mental development, failure to gain weight and grow (failure to thrive), poor feeding, lethargy, abnormal eye movements, short stature, breathing difficulties (apnoea or dyspnoea), malformations of the brain structures, and dysmorphic facial features, which can include slightly wide-set eyes, a depressed nasal bridge, thickening of the lips, large low-set ears and a prominent forehead.

Treatment for affected individuals aims to provide relief of any symptoms and support in the care of the individual. A high-fat, low-carbohydrate diet (so that most of the calories come from fats) can prevent the build-up of pyruvate that leads to acidosis. This means that the body uses energy from a different source, and although it will not cause any neurological improvements, it can help to reduce further damage. Some supplements may also be of benefit, as they are required for associated processes. These supplements may include thiamine, carnitine, coenzyme Q and lipoic acid, but they vary depending on the precise cause of the pyruvate dehydrogenase deficiency. If there are high levels of lactic acid in the body, fluids with electrolytes (sugars and salts) need to be given. Other medications may also be given to help to reduce the levels of lactic acid. Individuals who have a severe form of the disorder, who present shortly after birth, rarely survive beyond the first year.

Reviewed by Professor M Gardiner

Zellweger syndrome

Other names for this condition
- Bowen syndrome
- Cerebrohepatorenal syndrome
- ZS

Zellweger syndrome is a peroxisomal disorder, and is at the most severe end of the spectrum of peroxisomal biogenesis disorders.

Infants with this disorder present in the neonatal period with characteristic dysmorphic features that include a prominent forehead, large anterior fontanelle, broad nasal bridge, epicanthal folds, high arched palate, micrognathia, redundant neck skin folds, clinodactyly and talipes equinovarus. Neurological abnormalities are prominent, including severe hypotonia, areflexia, poor suck reflex and seizures. Neuronal migration defects may be observed on neuroimaging. Other features, such as corneal clouding, cataracts, pigmentary retinopathy, polycystic kidneys, cryptorchidism, dislocated hips and stippled epiphyses on radiographs (chondrodysplasia punctata) may be present. Liver disease is common, and includes hepatomegaly, conjugated hyperbilirubinaemia, progression to cirrhosis and liver failure in the first few months of life, but the hepatic involvement is overshadowed by the neurological symptoms. Failure of psychomotor development is evident in early infancy, and survival beyond 1 year is rare.

This disorder is genetically inherited from the parents in an autosomal recessive fashion.

The diagnosis of Zellweger syndrome is usually suspected clinically. The urine may show excess pipecolic acid, and medium- and long-chain dicarboxylic acids. The diagnosis of this disorder may be confirmed by establishing abnormalities in more than one peroxisomal function. Specific biochemical tests include very-long-chain fatty acids (VLCFAs), dihydroxyacetone phosphate acyltransferase activity, phytanate/pristanate levels and plasmalogens. Morphological studies of liver and/or skin for fibroblasts may show a complete absence of or reduced or abnormal structure of peroxisomes. The diagnosis is confirmed by specific enzyme analysis of skin fibroblasts.

There is no treatment for multiple-enzyme dysfunction, but supportive care with the administration of anticonvulsants, dietary supplements for the liver disease and muscle relaxants may be used. Bile-acid supplements may help to reduce cholestasis.

Reviewed by Dr M Cleary

Chapter 4

Lysosomal, sterol and lipid disorders

Lysosomal disorders

Lysosomes are intracellular organelles containing a large number of different enzymes at an acid pH, whose main function is the degradation of macromolecules. The lysosomal storage disorders are each caused by a specific enzyme deficiency resulting in abnormal storage of partially degraded macromolecules in the lysosomes.

The clinical spectrum of the storage disorders is wide, ranging from prenatal hydrops fetalis to mild disease in adulthood. Suggestive signs may include coarsening of facial features, neurological deterioration and hepatosplenomegaly. Patients with storage disorders often have a characteristic skeletal dysplasia (dysostosis multiplex) with a large skull, spinal deformities and short thick tubular bones. The liver and spleen are important sites for abnormal lysosomal storage, and consequently hepatosplenomegaly is a frequent finding, but the clinical picture is often dominated by neurodevelopmental regression.

Sterol disorders

Sterols are steroid alcohols, and they are found in fatty tissues. The most important sterols are cholesterol and some steroid hormones. Cholesterol is found on the outer membrane of cells and also in the bloodstream. It is obtained from dietary intake and is also produced by the liver. Steroid hormones affect the development and growth of the sex organs. They are usually derived from cholesterol in the reproductive organs and the adrenal glands. In sterol disorders the sterols can accumulate and cause a number of complications. They can have implications for the mental development of affected individuals.

Lipid disorders

Lipids, more commonly known as fats, are an important component of cell membranes and are stored in the body as an energy reserve. Lipid disorders are caused by a defect in certain enzymes that normally break down and process lipids so that the body can use them as an energy source. These defects can cause an accumulation of lipids, which is harmful to the organs of the body.

Anderson–Fabry disease

Other names for this condition
- Alpha-galactosidase A deficiency
- Fabry disease
- Angiokeratoma corporis diffusum
- Angiokeratoma diffuse
- Ceramide trihexosidase deficiency
- GLA deficiency

This disorder belongs to a group of conditions known as lysosomal storage disorders. In Anderson–Fabry disease there is a deficiency of the enzyme alpha-galactosidase A (ceramide trihexosidase), which results in the build-up of a fatty substance called globotriaosylceramide, in various organs.

This disorder is genetically inherited in an X-linked fashion.

Symptoms of Anderson–Fabry disease usually appear during childhood or adolescence. However, in some cases the onset has been reported to be delayed until the third decade. The early clinical features include a dark bluish-red rash (angiokeratoma), commonly seen in the bathing trunk area, umbilicus and the mucous membranes of the mouth, decreased sweating (hypohydrosis), and gastrointestinal manifestations such as alternating constipation and diarrhoea, abdominal pain and bloating. Slit-lamp examination of the eyes reveals haziness of the cornea (corneal dystrophy or cornea verticillata), which does not affect vision. Cataracts and tortuosity of the blood vessels in the retina can also be present. There are usually episodes of severe burning pain, known as acroparaesthesiae, in the hands and feet and sometimes in the arms and legs. Patients with Anderson–Fabry disease may also suffer from a sudden onset of sharp tingling pains in their fingers or toes, or experience acute abdominal pain, which is sometimes mistaken for an acute abdominal problem such as appendicitis. These episodes of sudden-onset pain are called Fabry crises. They may last for a few minutes but can sometimes last for days. They are usually brought on by fatigue, exercise, stress, fever or variations in temperature, and are often not relieved by standard painkillers. In addition, affected individuals may be intolerant of heat, which may lead to nausea, light-headedness, headaches and general weakness. Children with Anderson–Fabry disease often experience tiredness and lethargy, which affects their daily activities and school performance, and these symptoms are worsened by decreased sweating.

The life-threatening complications of Anderson–Fabry disease that are seen in adults, such as cardiac failure, thickening of the heart muscle, heart rhythm disturbances, end-stage kidney disease and strokes, are very rare in children. However, increased protein exrection in the urine, cardiac valve problems and MRI changes in the brain even without symptoms have been reported in older children and adolescents. The decrease in quality of life and the frequent episodes of pain may lead to depression and other behavioural changes. Other symptoms may include an accumulation of lymph within certain tissues, sometimes leading to lymphoedema.

Female patients who have symptoms of Anderson–Fabry disease vary in the degree to which they are affected by this condition. Some have mild symptoms and others are as severely affected as males. Any of the symptoms that affect male patients can be experienced by females, and can occur in childhood.

Some of the symptoms can be relieved with medication, including drugs to relieve pain in the hands and feet (gabapentin or carbamazepine). The gastrointestinal bloating and malabsorption symptoms that are seen in adults are sometimes relieved by pancreatic enzyme supplements. Later complications of the kidneys and heart may require specific treatment. Haemodialysis and kidney transplantation may be necessary in cases where kidney failure is prolonged. However, enzyme replacement therapy in which the missing enzyme is replaced by an intravenous infusion has recently become available in Europe and the USA. There are two orphan drugs that have been approved for use in the European Union, namely Fabrazyme® (produced by Genzyme) and Replagal® (produced by TKT). Genetic counselling is an important part of the management of this multi-system disorder.

Reviewed by Dr U Ramaswami

Batten disease – infantile form

Other names for this condition
- Batten disease – Finnish type
- Batten disease – Santavouri type
- INCL
- Infantile neuronal ceroid lipofuscinosis
- Santavouri disease
- Santavouri–Haltia disease

Batten disease consists of a group of disorders comprising four main clinical types as well as several other variant forms. In the infantile form, there is a build-up of lipofuscins, which are composed of fats and proteins, in the body. This form is caused by a deficiency of the palmitoyl protein thioesterase (PPT) enzyme, as a result of which, storage material known as granular osmiophilic deposits (GROD) accumulates in the brain and other body tissues, leading to severe deterioration.

This disorder is genetically inherited from the parents in an autosomal recessive fashion. Batten disease is more prevalent in populations of Scandinavian descent, particularly those with Finnish ancestry.

Symptoms in the infantile form usually begin to appear at approximately 1 year of age. The first signs of this disorder are convulsions and deterioration of mental and physical development. Affected individuals become increasingly unsteady when they are walking, develop low muscle tone and make involuntary jerky movements (ataxia). An abnormally small head (microcephaly) is obvious after approximately 1 to 2 years. Sight problems may be apparent, and these can progress to blindness by the age of 2 years. Individuals suffer from muscle jerks (myoclonic jerks), and in some cases characteristic rapid hand movements (more common in females) as if the child is knitting, which disappear within a few months. Other symptoms include excitability and behavioural problems.

In the third year of life, children are unable to control voluntary movements and may develop stiffened joints as well as joint and skeletal abnormalities. The joints may fuse in a closed position (flexion contractures), and there may be episodes during which the spine, neck and head are arched backwards (opisthotonos). Other symptoms include acne, puberty at an early age (precocious puberty), and the development of coarse hair on the face, chest, upper back or abdomen in females, due to excessive production of androgen. As this disorder is rapidly progressive, most children do not survive beyond 5 or 6 years of age, usually due to infections or other complications.

Treatment for this condition is symptomatic and supportive. If there are seizures, anticonvulsant medication may be of benefit. Physiotherapy and occupational therapy may help to maintain movement and muscle function. Continual optical care and the use of visual aids may help to support any visual disturbances. Research into the use of bone-marrow therapy as a treatment for this disorder is ongoing. Genetic counselling may be of benefit for individuals affected by this disorder.

Reviewed by Professor M Gardiner

Cystinosis

Other names for this condition
- Cystine storage disease
- Cystine transport protein, defect of
- Fanconi II
- Lignac–Fanconi syndrome

This disorder is caused by impaired transport of the amino acid cystine. Proteins are composed of a number of different amino acids, one of which is cystine. These proteins are broken down into amino acids in a specialised part of the cell called the lysosome, so that they can be reused by the body. Once the breakdown has occurred, cystine is normally transported out of the lysosome. In cystinosis, there is a problem with transporting the cystine out of the lysosome, which results in a build-up of cystine in this part of the cell. Because of its structure, cystine crystallises in all tissues, but the kidneys and the eyes are particularly affected.

This disorder is genetically inherited from the parents in an autosomal recessive fashion.

There are three clinical forms of cystinosis:

- infantile cystinosis
- juvenile or adolescent cystinosis
- adult or benign cystinosis.

In the infantile form of the disorder, symptoms usually appear during the first year of life, and include excessive thirst (polydipsia), the production of large amounts of urine (polyuria), episodes of dehydration often accompanied by a fever, and failure to grow and gain weight (failure to thrive). In some individuals there may also be bowing of the long bones, especially those of the legs, due to rickets. During infancy there may be a patchy loss of colour in the retina of the eye and increased sensitivity to light (photophobia), due to the accumulation of cystine crystals in the cornea. Kidney function becomes affected, and there is excessive loss of electrolytes (sodium, potassium and chloride as well as glucose, phosphate and amino acids) in the urine. This is the onset of renal Fanconi syndrome, which if untreated leads to kidney failure by 10 years of age. In addition, the thyroid gland may be affected, causing it to under-produce thyroxine.

In the juvenile form of cystinosis, symptoms may appear at any time between late childhood and adolescence. In individuals with this form of the disorder, cystine crystals are deposited in the cornea, causing sensitivity to light (photophobia). The kidneys are also affected, but not as severely as in the infantile form. However, progression to kidney failure still occurs. Some individuals develop rickets, with bowing of the long bones, especially those of the legs.

In the adult form of cystinosis, cystine crystals are normally found on the cornea and the conjunctiva of the eye during a routine eye test. In this form of the disorder, affected individuals may have crystalline deposits throughout the body, but they do not usually develop any kidney dysfunction. Most individuals show no symptoms, although a mild sensitivity to light may develop in middle age.

Treatment of this condition is symptomatic. Excessive loss of urine and electrolytes necessitates an increase in fluid and electrolyte intake. Supplementation with phosphate and vitamin D may help to prevent rickets. Mercaptamine (also known as Cystagon®) is a drug that lowers cystine levels within cells and which may delay or prevent kidney failure. Some individuals may still develop kidney failure and require a kidney transplant. Cysteamine eyedrops can dissolve the existing crystals and prevent the formation of further ones in the eyes. This will reduce the individual's sensitivity to light. If the thyroid gland is underactive, an oral dose of thyroxine may be given.

Reviewed by Dr G Besley

Fucosidosis

Other names for this condition

• Alpha-L-fucosidase deficiency

Fucosidosis is a rare inherited disorder that belongs to a group of conditions known as lysosomal storage disorders. It is caused by an absence or a deficiency of the enzyme alpha-L-fucosidase, which results in impaired fucosidase activity. Partially degraded chemicals that contain fucose remain in the body, accumulate and cause progressive damage to the cells. The defective gene (*FUCA1*) is located on the short arm of chromosome 1. Researchers believe that there are two types of this disorder, determined mainly by the severity of the symptoms.

Fucosidosis is genetically inherited from the parents in an autosomal recessive fashion.

The symptoms of fucosidosis vary widely, and affected individuals may not experience all of the symptoms described below. In general, symptoms do not appear until 6 to 18 months of age, although at birth the baby is larger than usual and will grow fast for the first few years of life. However, as the child ages, growth will be restricted. Affected individuals may show neurological and mental deterioration, which can lead to dementia and learning difficulties. Skin changes are also frequently observed. Known as angiokeratoma, these are small bright red nodules on the skin. Transverse purple lines on the nails have also been reported. Cold hands and feet are a common problem and do not respond to local heating.

Problems with bone formation and joint stiffness are common symptoms, a curve in the spine may be apparent, and the upper vertebrae and abnormally short neck are fragile. The chest may have an unusual shape, and is rigid and not as flexible as usual. Affected individuals may also have decreased muscle tension (hypotonia). The patient may walk with flexed knees and hips, and may also lose the ability to walk.

Other symptoms include an abnormally large heart, tongue, liver and spleen, and those affected may become prone to infections causing breathing problems. The tonsils may become enlarged and may need to be removed in order to clear the airway. Frequent ear infections may lead to hearing loss.

In some cases, affected individuals may have a characteristic facial appearance. The head may be larger than usual, with a prominent forehead. A broad nose with a flattened nasal bridge, large or low-set ears and coarse hair may also be apparent. Visual impairment is fairly common, and prominent blood vessels in the eye may be noticeable. Those affected may have thick skin, and can suffer from excessive perspiration and skin lesions. Individuals with this condition are unlikely to reach the first or second decade of life, depending on the severity of the condition.

Prenatal diagnosis is available through specialist tests. Treatment is mainly dependent upon symptoms. Bone-marrow transplantation has been performed in a few patients, with some promising early results. Anti-inflammatory drugs may help to relieve joint stiffness, and antibiotics may be administered to treat breathing problems. Fluid replacement may be considered in order to counter the excessive perspiration. Physiotherapy and hydrotherapy may be of benefit, and can improve general health and drain mucus from the chest. Caution is needed, as passive stretching may be painful. Genetic counselling is recommended for individuals affected by this condition.

Research into bone-marrow transplants and enzyme replacement therapy for treatment of this disorder is ongoing.

Reviewed by Dr C Hendriksz

Gaucher disease type 1

Other names for this condition

- Acid beta-glucosidase deficiency
- GBA deficiency
- GD 1
- Glucocerebrosidase deficiency
- Non-cerebral juvenile Gaucher disease

This is a disorder in which there is a deficiency of the enzyme glucocerebrosidase. This enzyme is found in lysosomes within specialised cells known as macrophages. The enzyme is responsible for breaking down a fatty substance called glucocerebroside into glucose and a fat called ceramide. Because of the enzyme deficiency, individuals with Gaucher disease type 1 (the commonest form of Gaucher disease) are unable to break down glucocerebroside, which accumulates inside the macrophages, so that they cannot function properly. When this happens, the macrophages are known as Gaucher cells. These are the main manifestation of the disorder, and are found in the bone marrow, the spleen and the liver.

This disorder is genetically inherited from the parents in an autosomal recessive fashion.

The symptoms vary from one individual to another. A minority of individuals have few or no symptoms (i.e. they are asymptomatic), whereas others are more seriously affected. Symptoms usually develop during adolescence, but may appear at any time from childhood to adulthood. An enlarged liver (hepatomegaly) and/or spleen (splenomegaly) is commonly the first symptom to be noticed. Other symptoms may include low levels of red blood cells (anaemia), which can lead to chronic fatigue, and low levels of platelets (thrombocytopenia). Platelets are important for the process of blood clotting, so a shortage of them can result in the affected individual bruising easily and having problems with bleeding. In female patients, prolonged bleeding episodes associated with menstruation are common. Skeletal abnormalities commonly occur, due to abnormal cells expanding and causing destruction of bone. This can result in intense pain, as well as degeneration, thinning and weakening of the bones (osteoporosis), which can lead to increased susceptibility to fractures and possibly deformity. Untreated patients may develop severe bone disease that requires multiple orthopaedic procedures. Occasionally there may also be involvement of the lungs and/or kidneys in individuals with this disorder. The incidence of Parkinson's disease is increased in adult patients who have Gaucher disease.

Enzyme replacement therapy using imiglucerase (Cerezyme®) and its predecessor, alglucerase (Ceredase®) has been developed and tested. These drugs have been shown to improve anaemia and low platelet levels. A decrease in the size of the liver and spleen and an improvement in skeletal symptoms have also been demonstrated. This effective therapy may limit or decrease the orthopaedic procedures necessary in treated patients. This is because the infused product can replace the missing enzyme. This medication is continued throughout life. Bone-marrow transplants have been given to individuals with Gaucher disease type 1, but the development of enzyme replacement therapy has superseded this treatment option. Bone-marrow transplants have been shown to be beneficial, but they require a matched donor and involve many risks that need to be taken into consideration. Zavesca® has been approved as an oral therapy for adults with mild to moderate Gaucher disease type 1 who are unable to have enzyme replacement therapy. This therapy improves the anaemia, the low platelet count and the bone disease. The size of the liver and spleen is also reduced, although the onset of action is slower than that achieved with enzyme replacement therapy.

Research into the use of L-cycloserine and N-butyl-deoxynojirimycin (NB–DNJ, Miglustat®), which are aimed at restricting the accumulation of Gaucher cells, is ongoing.

Reviewed by Dr C Hendriksz

GM2 gangliosidosis type 2 – infantile form

Other names for this condition

- Sandhoff disease
- Gangliosidosis beta-hexosaminidase deficiency
- GM2 gangliosidosis, O variant
- Hexosaminidase A and B deficiencies

In this disorder there is a deficiency of the hexosaminidase β-subunit. This subunit is required to form the enzymes hexosaminidase A and hexosaminidase B, which are needed to break down fatty materials known as GM2 gangliosides. If there is a deficiency or an absence of these enzymes, GM2 gangliosides will accumulate in the nerve cells of the brain and the organs of the body. This affects the ability of the central nervous system to function and leads to the symptoms of the condition. This disorder is very similar to Tay–Sachs disease (*see* p. 69), except that in the latter condition there is only a deficiency of hexosaminidase A.

This disorder is genetically inherited from the parents in an autosomal recessive fashion.

Symptoms of this form of the disorder commonly present during the first 6 months of life. Common symptoms include feeding problems, a generalised weakness and lethargy, an exaggerated startle reflex, an abnormal foot reflex (Babinski sign), enlargement of the spleen (splenomegaly) and/or the liver (hepatomegaly), a large head (macrocephaly) and seizures. There may be a delay in the development of physical and mental skills, and as the condition progresses there is a loss of previously acquired skills and an increase in muscle tension leading to permanent contraction of the muscles. During eye examination, affected individuals are frequently found to have a cherry-red spot at the back of the eye. There is generally a loss of vision that leads to blindness and a hearing loss that leads to deafness.

Treatment for affected individuals aims to provide relief of any symptoms and support in the care of the individual. Medication may be prescribed for seizures if these occur. The symptoms, severity and rate of progression of this condition vary from one individual to another. Children with this disorder rarely reach school age.

There are some early indications that Miglustat (Zavesca®) may be of some benefit in this disorder. Further research into the possibilities of stem-cell transplantation and gene-transfer therapy is ongoing.

Reviewed by Dr C Hendriksz

Lipodystrophy – Berardinelli–Seip syndrome

Other names for this condition
- Berardinelli–Seip lipodystrophy
- Brunzell syndrome
- Congenital generalised lipodystrophy
- Lipoatrophic diabetes
- Seip syndrome

This disorder belongs to a group of conditions known as lipodystrophies, in which there are abnormalities in the fatty (adipose) tissues of the body. There is a generalised, almost total loss of body fat, together with abnormalities in the metabolism of sugars and fats, and resistance to insulin (which controls blood sugar levels).

Berardinelli–Seip lipodystrophy is genetically transmitted by autosomal recessive inheritance.

Symptoms usually present soon after birth, and include a loss of fat beneath the skin (lipoatrophy), overdeveloped and prominent muscles (muscular hypertrophy), enlargement of the liver (hepatomegaly), and resistance to insulin (both natural and synthetic), which controls blood sugar levels, leading to diabetes mellitus. Other symptoms include darkening and thickening of patches of skin (acanthosis nigricans) and high levels of fats in the blood (hypertriglyceridaemia). There is commonly excessive production of a hormone that causes accelerated growth in height and precocious puberty in childhood, and in adults enlarged hands and feet (acromegaly), prominent ridges above the eyes (supraorbital ridges), enlargement of the upper or lower jaw (prognathism), and enlargement of the genitalia. Other symptoms that may occur in some individuals include excessive production of body hair (hirsutism), a delay in mental development, enlargement of the heart (hypertrophic cardiomyopathy), bone cysts, and a prominence of veins (phlebomegaly) in the upper and lower limbs. Acute inflammation of the pancreas (pancreatitis) may also occur.

Affected individuals may have a large appetite because their utilisation of energy is inefficient. Dietary treatment with an emphasis on modest frequent meals and a low fat intake is beneficial. Some individuals undergo cosmetic surgery to restore normal facial features. The life expectancy of individuals with this condition frequently does not extend beyond middle age, due to kidney and liver problems and cardiomyopathy.

Reviewed by Dr PH Robinson

Mucopolysaccharidosis type 2

Other names for this condition
- Iduronate-2-sulphatase deficiency
- Hunter disease
- Hunter syndrome

Mucopolysaccharidosis type 2 is a lysosomal disorder. Lysosomes are intracellular organelles that contain a large number of different enzymes whose main function is to break down macromolecules. Each of the lysosomal storage disorders is due to a specific enzyme deficiency resulting in abnormal storage of partially degraded macromolecules in the lysosomes.

The mucopolysaccharidoses (MPS) are a group of progressive multi-system disorders that affect the bones and joints, the brain, the liver, the spleen and the upper airways. They can be grouped according to the underlying enzyme deficiency. In MPS 2 the underlying enzyme defect is iduronate-2-sulphatase deficiency, which leads to an accumulation of partially degraded macromolecules known as glycosaminoglycans in the lysosome, and causes cellular dysfunction.

Hunter syndrome is inherited as an X-linked disorder.

The earliest symptoms are often non-specific, such as recurrent ear infections or noisy breathing due to upper airway obstruction. Other signs are recurrent inguinal and umbilical hernias and coarse facial features. The onset of symptoms and signs in Hunter syndrome occurs between 2 and 4 years of age. Persistent otitis media can cause reduced hearing, and speech delay is a common occurrence. Skeletal involvement is the norm, with joint stiffness and deformity. Other symptoms and signs include diarrhoea, an enlarged liver (hepatomegaly) and short stature. In contrast to many other MPS conditions, corneal clouding is not usual in Hunter syndrome, but retinal degeneration is a complication. The accumulation of glycosaminoglycans can lead to compression of the cervical spinal cord. The condition can also affect the heart, causing cardiac valvular disease and cardiomyopathy. Anaesthesia should be undertaken with care in children with mucopolysaccharidosis type 2, as they are difficult to intubate due to MPS deposition around the airway. Intubation is further compromised by the vulnerability of the cervical spinal cord, and should only be undertaken in a specialist centre.

Broadly speaking, there are two categories of Hunter syndrome – those cases involving the brain, in which there is a neurodegenerative pattern of disease, and those in whom intellectual progress is normal or near normal. This distinction can be difficult to make in early childhood. Whereas the severe form progresses to immobility and loss of skills, with death in the early teenage years, individuals with the non-neurological form survive to adulthood. However, cardiorespiratory complications limit their lifespan in adulthood.

The widespread nature of the effects of MPS means that management requires the coordination of the input of many specialists by a paediatrician with expertise in this field. The specialists would include those with expertise in cardiology, neurosurgery, ENT, physiotherapy and orthopaedics.

Recent developments in treatment have led to successful human trials of enzyme replacement therapy for this disorder. This therapy is not expected to cross the blood–brain barrier, and therefore will not treat the cerebral aspects of the disease. However, the systemic features respond to intravenous enzyme replacement therapy.

The condition is diagnosed by detection of elevated levels of glycosaminoglycans in the urine and by specific enzyme determination in white cells. Prenatal diagnosis is possible. Mutation studies may determine the underlying mutation, which is of help in determining carrier status.

Genetic counselling should be offered in order to detect carriers within the family.

Reviewed by Dr M Cleary

Niemann–Pick disease – type A

> **Other names for this condition**
> - Lipidosis, sphingomyelin
> - NPD
> - Sphingomyelinase deficiency
> - Sphingomyelin lipidosis

This condition belongs to the Niemann–Pick group of disorders, in which the breakdown of a particular type of fatty acid, called sphingomyelin, is impaired. There are thought to be up to six forms in this group of disorders – types A to F – each with distinctive characteristics. Type A is the commonest form, and it presents in infants and young children. It is characterised by enlargement of the liver (hepatomegaly) and/or spleen (splenomegaly), often with jaundice and anaemia, and other symptoms include poor feeding, failure to thrive and severe developmental delay, with loss of learned skills. There is a deficiency of the enzyme known as acid sphingomyelinase (ASM), which is required to break down sphingomyelin, a fatty substance that occurs in all types of cells. As a result, sphingomyelin accumulates in certain organs of the body. Niemann–Pick disease is more common in people of Ashkenazi Jewish descent.

This disorder occurs as a result of autosomal recessive inheritance.

In Niemann–Pick disease – type A, sphingomyelin accumulation begins during fetal development in the womb, and occurs mainly in the liver, spleen and brain. Symptoms begin to appear within the first few months following birth. These may include difficulties with feeding, apathy, and failure to thrive. There may be distension of the abdomen caused by enlargement of the liver and/or spleen (hepatosplenomegaly), and also yellowing of the eyes and skin (jaundice). Accumulation of sphingomyelin in the brain and nervous system causes loss of muscle tone. There is progressive loss of acquired skills such as head control, the ability to sit, and the ability to hold and handle toys. Seizures may occur. In many cases, examination with an ophthalmoscope reveals a cherry-red spot at the back of the eye. This is seen because the part of the eye known as the macula, which is covered by few nerve fibres, contrasts in colour with the rest of the retina, which is pale because of the accumulating sphingolipids. The range of symptoms varies from one individual to another, but the severity of the symptoms increases throughout the course of the disease. Children with this disorder rarely survive beyond 5 years of age.

The disorder is diagnosed by demonstration of reduced or absent enzyme activity in white blood cells and fibroblasts cultured from skin. Prenatal diagnosis and screening for carriers are available. Treatment for individuals with Niemann–Pick disease aims to provide relief of any symptoms and support in the care of the child. Genetic counselling may be of benefit to individuals affected by this disorder.

Reviewed by Dr PH Robinson

Tay–Sachs disease – infantile form

Other names for this condition

- Amaurotic familial idiocy
- Amaurotic familial infantile idiocy
- Cerebromacular degeneration
- GM2 gangliosidosis, type 1
- Hexosaminidase α-subunit deficiency (variant B)
- Infantile cerebral ganglioside storage
- Lipidosis, ganglioside infantile
- Sphingolipidosis, Tay–Sachs
- Tay–Sachs type 1

In this disorder there is a deficiency of the enzyme hexosaminidase A, which is required to break down fatty substances known as gangliosides. If this enzyme is absent or deficient, these GM2 gangliosides accumulate in the nerve cells and the brain. This affects the ability of the central nervous system to function, and leads to the symptoms of the condition. This form of Tay–Sachs disease is also referred to as the classical form.

This disorder is genetically inherited from the parents in an autosomal recessive fashion. It is more common in Jews of Ashkenazi descent.

Symptoms of this condition usually present between 3 and 6 months after birth. They include a loss of previously acquired skills such as smiling, crawling and the ability to grasp or reach out to objects, or to sit or hold the head up. There is also a loss of muscle tone (hypotonia), an exaggerated startle response to sudden noises, listlessness, and eye examination reveals a cherry-red spot at the back of the eye. As the disorder progresses, there is a gradual loss of vision and hearing, affected individuals find it difficult to swallow, and muscle stiffness develops which leads to restricted movements and eventually paralysis. There is enlargement of the head (macrocephaly), fits (seizures) start to occur, and there is a progressive loss of intellectual abilities.

Treatment for affected individuals aims to provide relief of any symptoms and support in the care of the individual. Medication may be prescribed for seizures if these occur. Those affected rarely survive beyond the age at which they start school.

Reviewed by Dr G Besley

Chapter 5

Carbohydrate and glycosylation disorders

Carbohydrate disorders

Carbohydrate disorders are caused by a defect in or an absence of one of the enzymes that break down certain sugars so that they can be absorbed by the body. An example of this is sucrose (also known as table sugar), which has two components, glucose and fructose. When a person consumes sucrose, the body breaks it down into glucose and fructose. This also applies to carbohydrates in foods such as pasta or bread, which are composed of longer chains of sugar molecules. A defect in the enzyme that controls the breakdown of sugars means that sugar accumulates in the body because it has not been absorbed. This build-up causes the symptoms associated with these disorders.

Glycosylation disorders

The *congenital disorders of glycosylation (CDGs)*, formerly known as *carbohydrate-deficient glycoprotein syndromes*, are a group of disorders that are caused by problems with adding sugar chains (oligosaccharides) to proteins to form glycoproteins, a process known as glycosylation. Glycoproteins are needed by the body for a number of different functions. They maintain growth and aid blood coagulation as well as playing a part in the functioning of all tissues and organs. In this group of disorders, there is a deficiency of a specific enzyme that plays a role in glycosylation, as a result of which glycosylation cannot be performed properly, and this has an effect on various systems. Most of the CDGs are caused by defects in the N-linked oligosaccharides (N-glycans). These types of sugar chains are needed by the body for protein stability and cell communication. A defect can lead to problems with the body's organs and other complications.

Congenital disorders of glycosylation – type Ia

Other names for this condition

- Carbohydrate-deficient glycoprotein syndrome – type Ia
- CDG type Ia
- Disorders of N-glycan processing – type Ia
- Phosphomannomutase deficiency
- PMM deficiency

This condition is one of a group of disorders in which there are abnormal oligosaccharides (sugar chains). This is due to a deficiency or an absence of an enzyme known as phosphomannomutase. The oligosaccharides attach to proteins to form glycoproteins. Glycoproteins have several important functions, including signalling how cells in the body interact with one another, aiding the transfer of nutrients around the body, playing a part in the coagulation of blood, and acting as hormones that regulate certain activities or organs in the body. Because the oligosaccharides are abnormal in this condition, the functions of the glycoproteins are affected, and this results in the symptoms of carbohydrate-deficient glycoprotein syndrome.

This condition is inherited in an autosomal recessive fashion.

Symptoms usually appear shortly after birth. In the infantile stage of the disorder, they commonly include feeding problems, including vomiting and diarrhoea, which can lead to failure to gain weight and grow (failure to thrive), as well as a delay in physical and mental development and a loss of muscle tone (hypotonia). There may also be an enlarged liver (hepatomegaly), dysfunction of the liver, inverted nipples, abnormal distribution of fat pads, and squinting. Certain parts of the brain may be underdeveloped (olivopontocerebellar atrophy), and there may be a collection of fluid in the sac that surrounds the heart (pericardial effusion), disease of the heart muscle (cardiomyopathy) and restricted movement of some of the joints of the limbs. Other symptoms include crossed eyes (esotropia), seizures and a tendency to have problems with bleeding. Other organs may also be affected.

In late infancy and childhood, affected individuals commonly develop slurred speech, an inability to coordinate muscle movements (ataxia), and a delay in intellectual development. Seizures and stroke-like episodes may be triggered by fevers or infection. In addition, some of the cells in the retina of the eye may become overactive in producing the pigmentation, resulting in damage to the photoreceptor cells (retinitis pigmentosa). During the teenage years most of the medical problems stabilise, but any skeletal abnormalities may become noticeable. These can include short stature, curving of the spine (scoliosis) and loss of bone density (osteopenia). There may also be further weakening of the muscles of the legs. In adulthood, problems related to the reproductive system become apparent. Males tend to pass through puberty later than normal, and females may have multiple hormonal problems during puberty. Most individuals with this condition are unable to live independently in adulthood.

Treatment for affected individuals aims to provide relief of any symptoms and support in the care of the individual. Feeding may be helped by using a tube that is passed through the nose into the stomach (nasogastric tube), as well as by using supplements that are high in calories. A wide range of specialists may need to be consulted, including those with expertise in paediatrics, neurology, ophthalmology, orthopaedics, endocrinology and haematology. Physiotherapy, speech therapy and the aid of a dietitian may be of benefit.

Reviewed by Dr C Hendriksz

Fanconi–Bickel syndrome

Other names for this condition

- Hepatorenal glycogenosis with renal Fanconi syndrome
- Hepatic glycogenosis with Fanconi nephropathy
- Hepatic glycogenosis with aminoaciduria and glucosuria
- Fanconi syndrome with intestinal malabsorption and galactose intolerance
- FBS
- Glycogenosis, Fanconi type
- Glycogen storage disease XI
- Pseudo-phlorizin diabetes

Symptoms of this disorder present in infancy and include failure to grow or gain weight (failure to thrive), enlargement of the liver (hepatomegaly) and failure of the bones to harden due to a deficiency of phosphate (hypophosphataemic rickets). Other symptoms include a protruding abdomen, enlarged kidneys, growth defects and decreased bone calcification, decreased bone density or reduced bone mass (osteopenia). Long periods of time without food may cause mild low blood sugar and raised levels of ketone bodies in the body tissues. Findings include the presence of high levels of lipids in the blood (hyperlipidaemia), massive excretion of glucose in the urine (glucosuria), high levels of protein in the urine (proteinuria) and abnormal urinary excretion of phosphate (hyperphosphaturia) and bicarbonate (renal tubular acidosis or RTA). Other findings include the presence of amino acids in the urine (aminoaciduria) and usually a high level of organic acids, lactate, ketone bodies and carnitine in the urine. The *GLUT2* gene may be expressed in the liver, kidneys, pancreas and intestines.

This disorder may be suspected if hypergalactosaemia is discovered. A few cases of Fanconi–Bickel syndrome have been diagnosed by newborn screening programmes. In the past, most patients have been detected because high levels of glucose were present in the urine (mimicking diabetes). Treatment for individuals with this disease aims to provide relief of any symptoms and support in the care of the individual. Treatment may include phosphate, bicarbonate and 1,25-dihydroxy vitamin D. Night-time cornstarch and daytime fructose-containing carbohydrate supplements may also be of benefit. A balanced diet with frequent feedings is recommended.

Reviewed by Professor GT Berry

Fructose intolerance – hereditary

Other names for this condition
- Fructose-1-phosphate aldolase deficiency
- Fructose aldolase B deficiency
- Fructosaemia
- HFI

Hereditary fructose intolerance is an inherited disorder that is characterised by the inability to digest fructose (a natural fruit sugar used in foods, including many baby foods) or sucrose (cane sugar or brown sugar). This intolerance is due to a deficiency of an enzyme known as fructose-1-phosphate aldolase, which results in a build-up of fructose-1-phosphate in the kidney, liver and small intestine. The gene responsible for this disorder is located on the long arm of chromosome 9.

This disorder is genetically inherited from the parents in an autosomal recessive fashion.

Symptoms of hereditary fructose intolerance develop after fructose has been added to the diet of affected individuals, and include poor feeding as a baby, jaundice, prolonged vomiting, severe abdominal pain, low blood sugar (hypoglycaemia) and failure to grow or gain weight (failure to thrive). The formation of fibrous structures in the liver tissue can affect the function of the liver, there may also be enlargement of the liver and spleen (hepatosplenomegaly), and a few children will go on to develop liver disease. There may also be bleeding in the stomach and intestines due to impaired functioning of clotting factors. Increased levels of fructose have been found in the blood and urine and decreased levels of glucose and phosphate have been found in the blood. Individuals affected by this disorder may also experience irritability, prolonged crying, excessive sleepiness and diarrhoea, and there may be a yellowish colouring in the eyes (icterus). Many affected children develop a strong distaste for sweet foods due to their association with experiencing the symptoms. Prolonged fructose ingestion in infants leads to renal failure and death, so it is essential to obtain an early diagnosis and then eliminate fructose and sucrose from the diet. This disorder may cause stunting of growth and nutritional failure with kidney calcification in adolescents and young adults.

In the past, diagnosis was made at birth either by a fructose tolerance test or by a liver biopsy. As both of these tests are associated with a high risk to a newborn baby, DNA testing for this condition is increasingly being recommended, and now provides the means of definitive diagnosis in the majority of patients without the need for invasive biopsies. Urine tests can detect fructose in the urine and blood tests can detect increased levels of liver enzymes in the blood. Early diagnosis and a fructose- and sucrose-free diet are important in order to avoid physical damage and enable the child, adolescent or young adult to lead a normal life. Vitamin C and folic acid should be supplemented, and the prescription should be sugar-free. Genetic counselling may be of benefit to individuals affected by this disorder.

Reviewed by Professor T Cox

Galactosaemia

Other names for this condition
- Classical galactosaemia
- GALT deficiency
- Galactose-1-phosphate uridyl transferase deficiency

Galactose is a sugar that is a constituent of lactose (the form of sugar found in milk, including breast milk, and in the majority of infant milk formulas). Use of the term galactosaemia (increased levels of galactose in the blood) usually refers to 'classical' galactosaemia and its synonyms listed above. (Blood levels of galactose may also be increased in two other conditions, namely galactokinase deficiency and UDP-galactose-4-epimerase deficiency. Galactokinase deficiency is a rare cause of cataract in children who are otherwise completely normal. Galactose-4-epimerase deficiency may be harmless if it affects only blood cells, but a generalised form causes vomiting and jaundice in the newborn, deafness, severe developmental delay and cataract in a minority of cases.)

In classical galactosaemia, the body's ability to convert galactose into glucose is impaired. Galactose-1-phosphate, derived from galactose, builds up in the body and becomes toxic. This disorder is caused by a deficiency of a liver enzyme known as galactose-1-phosphate uridyl transferase (GALT). This enzyme is coded for by the *GALT* gene, which is located on the short arm of chromosome 9.

This disorder is inherited in an autosomal recessive fashion.

Early symptoms of this disorder in babies within a few days of birth include poor feeding, vomiting, poor weight gain, jaundice and an enlarged liver (hepatomegaly). Older infants with this disorder who have not been recognised and treated show irritability, listlessness, cataracts, liver failure and kidney damage. Other symptoms may include low blood sugar (hypoglycaemia) and reduced growth of the head. Severe *E. coli* infections are common in untreated infants, and can be life threatening. Early recognition and treatment permit complete resolution of cataract and liver disease, but for reasons that are not known there is a reduction in the expected IQ, and impairment of verbal and speech skills, which do not appear to respond to current treatment methods. There is late or absent puberty and impaired function of the ovaries in female individuals. Puberty and fertility in males are not affected. Older patients may experience unsteadiness and lack of muscular coordination (ataxia), as well as difficulties with direction finding.

In some countries this disorder is screened for as part of a newborn screening programme for congenital disorders. Depending on the screening methods used, the enzyme itself (GALT) or the concentration of galactose in the blood may be measured. The finding of GALT deficiency will confirm classical galactosaemia. Measurement of galactose levels will detect cases of galactokinase deficiency and epimerase deficiency as well as classical galactosaemia. The finding of excess galactose in the blood should be followed by measurement of GALT activity. Galactokinase deficiency and epimerase deficiency must be considered if GALT activity is normal in an infant with elevated galactose levels.

Children with this disorder should follow a strict galactose- and lactose-free diet. This is achieved by excluding all milk products and all known sources of galactose from the diet. Medicines containing lactose should also be avoided. Girls with galactosaemia may require oestrogen replacement therapy to induce and maintain sexual development around the normal time of puberty. There is a high risk of infertility due to underdevelopment of the ovaries.

Reviewed by Dr P Robinson

Glucose transporter type 1 deficiency

Other names for this condition
- De Vivo disease
- Glucose transporter protein syndrome
- Glucose transporter type 1 deficiency syndrome
- GLUT1 deficiency
- GLUT1-DS

Glucose transporter type 1 deficiency is a rare disorder characterised by infantile seizures, developmental delay and learning disabilities. Glucose transporters are components of glycoproteins, which are involved in transporting glucose to most cells in the body. This disorder is caused by defects on the glucose transporter type 1 deficiency gene (*SLC2A1*) that encodes the Glut-1 protein. This gene is located on the short arm of chromosome 1.

The disorder is inherited in an autosomal dominant fashion.

Symptoms of glucose transporter type 1 deficiency are not present at birth and do not usually appear until infancy. They include low glucose levels in the cerebrospinal fluid that surrounds the brain and spinal cord (hypoglycorrhachia), a small head (microcephaly), involuntary uncoordinated movements (ataxia), erratic eye movements such as rolling of the eyes (opsoclonus), unclear pronunciation of words (dysarthia), decreased muscle tone (hypotonia), movement and posture abnormalities and paralysis of one side (hemiparesis) or both sides of the body. Other symptoms in children include inactivity and unresponsiveness, sometimes verging on unconsciousness, a hypnotic-like trance (somnolence), confusion, epilepsy, sleep disturbances and recurrent headaches.

Diagnosis of glucose transporter type 1 deficiency is made on the basis of clinical tests. As the disorder is not apparent at birth, prenatal diagnosis is not usually available. Treatment of this disorder includes a ketogenic diet in which most carbohydrates are replaced by fats and proteins. This diet has been reported to help control seizures. Individuals affected by this disorder are recommended to avoid certain drugs, namely barbiturates and methylxanthines. Methylxanthines are found in coffee and other caffeine-related products. Genetic counselling is recommended.

Reviewed by Dr CA Davies

Glycogen storage disease type III

Other names for this condition
- Amylo-1,6-glucosidase deficiency
- Cori disease
- Debrancher deficiency
- Glycogen storage disease III
- Glycogenosis type III
- Limit dextrinosis

This disorder belongs to a group known as the glycogen storage diseases (GSDs) in which there is a deficiency in an enzyme that is required to break down glycogen compounds into simple sugars known as monosaccharides. This enzyme deficiency causes an accumulation of glycogen in the tissues where, due to the defect in the enzyme, the body is unable to produce sufficient amounts of glucose in the blood stream and cannot use glucose as a source of energy.

The severe forms of GSDs are characterised by the reduced ability to store energy as glycogen inbetween meal times or during exercise, which results in low blood glucose (hypoglycaemia), which is very common. In type III the missing enzyme is amylo-1 6 glucosidase otherwise known as the debrancher enzyme.

Glycogen storage disease III is genetically inherited from the parents in an autosomal recessive fashion.

This disorder is characterised by the presence of abnormally high levels of glycogen in the liver and the muscles. This usually leads to enlargement of the liver (hepatomegaly), which causes the abdomen to protrude. The muscles are weaker than usual and there tends to be decreased muscle tone (hypotonia). Commonly there are low blood sugar levels (hypoglycaemia) and high levels of fatty substances (hyperlipaemia). In some cases there may be weakening of the heart, with thickening of the heart muscles (cardiomyopathy). Individuals with this disorder tend to have short stature, and puberty may be delayed, although normal adult height is usually reached. Some affected individuals have few symptoms, usually just an enlarged liver and a protruding abdomen, whereas others have more problems. Symptoms in this disorder may progress with age. It is possible that some individuals with this disorder show no symptoms.

Glycogen storage disease type III can be diagnosed by means of blood tests, and in rare cases liver and muscle biopsies are needed. Treatment aims to prevent low blood sugar levels (hypoglycaemia) by giving frequent small carbohydrate-based meals that are high in protein. A gastric or nasogastric tube may be needed overnight, or alternatively cornstarch supplements may be given to provide an energy source and prevent hypoglycaemia during this period. A normal lifespan is expected in individuals with this disorder, although there may be worsening of the muscle symptoms, and cardiac disease may develop with age. Genetic counselling may be of benefit to individuals affected by this disorder.

Reviewed by Professor J Leonard

Glycogen synthase deficiency

Other names for this condition

- Glycogenosis type 0
- GSD-0
- Glycogen storage disease type 0
- Liver glycogen synthase deficiency

Glycogen synthase deficiency is a rare genetic disorder characterised by low blood sugar levels and abnormally high levels of acidic substances known as ketones in the blood and urine. This disorder is caused by a deficiency of the liver enzyme glycogen synthetase, which leads to low glycogen levels in the liver. The defective gene that codes for the enzyme is known as *GYS2*, and is located on the long arm of chromosome 12.

The disorder is genetically inherited from the parents in an autosomal recessive fashion.

Symptoms of this disorder include drowsiness, uncoordinated eye movements, growth delay, lethargy, nausea, vomiting, headache, low muscle tone (hypotonia), seizures, visual problems and coma. Those affected also show signs of lack of interest, morning fatigue, disorientation, seizures, abnormal levels of perspiration, pale or grey skin (pallor), rapid heartbeat (tachycardia), speech problems and mental confusion. In addition, the liver may be slightly enlarged. Many of these symptoms may be due to low blood sugar levels (hypoglycaemia), which occur before breakfast or during long periods without food.

Diagnosis is made by a liver biopsy and other clinical tests. Treatment includes consulting a dietitian about management of the patient's diet. The diet should consist of adequate proteins and calories to aid growth. Those affected should eat frequently and avoid going for long periods without food. Uncooked cornstarch is recommended, as it releases glucose slowly. Studies have shown that dietary treatment over 1 year, which includes frequent meals that are high in protein and low in carbohydrate, improves growth and relieves the symptoms of hypoglycaemia. Genetic counselling may be of benefit to individuals affected by this condition.

Reviewed by Dr MJ Henderson

Hyperinsulinism–hypoglycaemia

Other names for this condition
- Congenital hyperinsulinism
- Familial hyperinsulinism
- HI
- Hyperinsulinaemic hypoglycaemia
- Islet dysregulation syndrome
- Pancreatic nesidioblastosis
- Persistent hyperinsulinaemic hypoglycaemia of infancy
- PHHI

Hyperinsulinism–hypoglycaemia is a rare disorder that is characterised by abnormally high levels of insulin and low blood sugar levels (hypoglycaemia). The disorder is due to the pancreas producing too much insulin. This causes persistent low blood sugar levels, which can result in seizures, brain damage and, in some cases, death. The commonest type of severe hyperinsulinism–hypoglycaemia occurs in individuals with diabetes type 1 who take insulin.

This disorder can be genetically inherited from the parents in an autosomal recessive fashion. In some cases it is inherited in an autosomal dominant manner.

The symptoms of this disorder vary according to the age of the individual and the severity of the hypoglycaemia. The main symptoms are due to the effects of the lack of glucose on the brain or on the autonomic nervous system, which is the part of the nervous system that is responsible for control of the involuntary muscles (e.g. bladder, bowel). Symptoms in infants include respiratory distress and breathing difficulties, lethargy, hypothermia, irritability, feeding difficulties, seizures, heart problems (tachycardia), shaking, and blue discoloration of the skin due to a lack of oxygen in the blood (cyanosis). Older children may show different symptoms, including behaviour problems, lack of attention, anxiety, headache, lethargy, nausea, seizures and loss of consciousness. Other symptoms in older children include sweating, shaking, heart problems, hypothermia, vomiting, hunger and increased appetite. Affected individuals may also stare and squint due to eye abnormalities.

In many cases the symptoms can be reversed when glucose levels are returned to normal. However, children who have prolonged or recurrent hyperinsulism–hypoglycaemia are at risk of brain damage and developmental delay.

Early diagnosis and treatment are essential in order to prevent seizures and brain damage. Treatment may involve the use of medications to reduce insulin secretion or to stimulate glucose release. A change in diet to include more carbohydrates may be recommended in order to increase glucose levels, and a gastrostomy tube may be used to feed infants who are unable to tolerate an increase in glucose. Partial or total surgical removal of the pancreas (pancreatectomy) may be undertaken in infants who fail to respond to other medical treatments.

Reviewed by Professor PM Stewart

Sucrase isomaltase deficiency

Other names for this condition
- Congenital sucrose intolerance
- Congenital sucrase–isomaltase deficiency
- Sucrose isomaltose malabsorption
- CSID
- Disaccharide intolerance I
- SI deficiency

Sucrase isomaltase deficiency is a rare disorder characterised by a deficiency or absence of sucrase and isomaltase enzyme activity in the gastrointestinal tract. Sucrose (table sugar) and isomaltase (a form of starch) cannot be broken down and absorbed. As a result, undigested sugars remain in the intestine and are fermented in the colon, causing diarrhoea. At least five types of sucrase isomaltase deficiency have been documented.

The gene responsible for sucrase isomaltase deficiency is thought to be located on the short arm of chromosome 3. This disorder is genetically inherited from the parents in an autosomal recessive fashion.

Symptoms of sucrase isomaltase deficiency become evident in breastfed babies when sucrose, which is found in some solid foods, fruit juices and some medications, is introduced to their diet. In formula-fed infants, symptoms will appear earlier if the formula milk contains sucrose or polycose. In some cases symptoms may not present until puberty. Symptoms vary according to the individual, and may improve as the child gets older. They include watery diarrhoea, abdominal swelling, discomfort and flatulence. Severely affected infants may show lack of growth and weight gain (failure to thrive), due to the malabsorption of nutrients. Other symptoms include irritability, colic, vomiting, dehydration, irritation of the skin on the buttocks, and excess acid in the blood (acidosis). Kidney stones may also be associated with this disorder.

Sucrase isomaltase deficiency is diagnosed on the basis of a clinical evaluation, a detailed patient history, and specialised tests, including blood and urine tests. Faeces may show increased amounts of sucrose, glucose and fructose, and an acid pH below 5. Enzyme tests can be used to measure the activity of sucrase isomaltase in the intestines. A sucrose hydrogen breath test reveals abnormally high levels of hydrogen in the breath of affected individuals after they have ingested sucrose. Sucrase isomaltase deficiency can sometimes be misdiagnosed as irritable bowel syndrome, food allergy, cystic fibrosis, coeliac disease or Williams syndrome.

Treatment includes dietary management with a low-sucrose or sucrose-free diet. A starch-free or low-starch diet may also be advised in the early years of life. In addition, vitamin supplements may be recommended. Some of those affected may benefit from yeast-derived invertase, which exhibits sucrase activity and is taken orally with food. Commercial enzyme replacement therapy is available in the form of the orphan drug Sacrosidase (Sucraid®). This has been approved by the Food and Drug Administration in the USA.

Reviewed by Dr PH Robinson

Uridine diphosphate galactose-4-epimerase deficiency

Other names for this condition
- UDP-galactose-4-epimerase deficiency
- GALE deficiency

Galactose is a sugar found in lactose-containing foods such as milk and other dairy products. It is broken down in the gut to form glucose and galactose. Galactose is further broken down in the body by a series of chemical reactions, each of which requires a specific enzyme. There are three recognised inborn errors of galactose metabolism:

- galactose-1-phosphate uridyltransferase (GALT) deficiency – classical galactosaemia
- galactokinase deficiency
- uridine diphosphate galactose-4-epimerase (GALE) deficiency.

All the disorders of galactose metabolism are inherited in an autosomal recessive manner.

GALE is a very rare form of galactosaemia, much less common than classical galactosaemia. It occurs in both mild and severe forms. Affected individuals with the severe form have symptoms similar to those of classical galactosaemia, with vomiting, failure to thrive, jaundice and liver disease in the newborn period. These symptoms improve when galactose is excluded from the diet. The full impact of this disorder in the long term remains unclear, as it has only been recognised in a few families. For example, some affected individuals have had facial dysmorphism and deafness, but it is not yet known whether these features can be attributed to GALE deficiency. Similarly, it is uncertain whether other complications seen in classical galactosaemia, such as ovarian dysfunction, occur in GALE deficiency. The milder form of GALE deficiency appears to be a benign disorder.

The diagnosis is made by investigating the clinical features described above, or by newborn screening. Biochemical tests show the typical findings of galactosaemia, namely abnormal liver function tests, low blood glucose levels and increased excretion of amino acids in the urine. Galactose may be present in the urine, where it is detected as positive reducing substances. Since classical galactosaemia is more common, normal GALT enzyme activity should be established before suspecting GALE deficiency. GALE enzyme activity can be measured in red blood cells. Prenatal diagnosis is possible.

Treatment of severe GALE deficiency involves management with a low-galactose diet. In contrast to GALT deficiency, a small amount of galactose is usually administered in order to allow production of galactoproteins and galactolipids.

Reviewed by Dr M Cleary

Chapter 6

Purine, pyrimidine and porphyria disorders

A purine is any of a group of organic compounds that are found in tissues, the two major purines being adenine and guanine. Others include uric acid, xanthine and hypoxanthine.

A pyrimidine is any of a group of organic compounds that are found in certain coenzymes and in tissues, the three major pyrimidines being thymine, uracil and cytosine.

Both purines and pyrimidines are components of DNA. They are involved in a number of processes, each of which is catalysed by a different enzyme. When there is a deficiency of one of these enzymes it causes disorders that can affect many of the body systems, particularly the kidneys.

Porphyrias

The porphyrias are a group of seven disorders. These are as follows:

- acute intermittent porphyria (AIP)
- aminolevulinate dehydratase deficiency porphyria (ADP)
- congenital porphyria (CP)
- cutanea tarda porphyria (PCT)
- erythropoietic protoporphyria (EEP)
- hereditary coproporphyria (HCP)
- variegate porphyria (VP).

Many of the porphyrias are inherited, and a number of them are acquired. Each is caused by a defect in a gene that codes for one of the seven enzymes that convert aminolevulinic acid (ALA) into haem. Haem is used in molecules that carry oxygen for use in the cells (e.g. haemoglobin in the red blood cells). In each type of porphyria a specific enzyme is deficient, and this causes the porphyrins to accumulate.

Acute intermittent porphyria

Other names for this condition

- AIP
- Swedish porphyria

This disorder belongs to a group of conditions known as the porphyrias. In this particular disorder there is a deficiency of the enzyme porphobilinogen deaminase, which slows the conversion into haem and leads to a build-up of aminolevulinic acid (ALA) and porphobilinogen (PBG), the latter being produced directly from ALA. This can cause acute attacks that affect the nervous system.

Acute intermittent porphyria does *not* cause any skin symptoms in sunlight, unlike most of the other porphyrias.

The disorder is inherited in an autosomal dominant fashion.

Affected individuals usually develop symptoms after they have reached puberty. However, many people who inherit the gene for this condition do not display any symptoms at all.

The main symptom of an acute attack is abdominal pain (or sometimes back pain), and this can be accompanied by nausea, vomiting, constipation, confusion and hallucinations. The urine may be red or brownish (particularly if left to stand for testing), due to an excess of porphyrins. The salt content of the blood may fall (hyponatraemia), and a blood test is needed to check whether this needs to be treated. There may also be pain in the arms and legs, a rapid heartbeat, increased blood pressure, muscle weakness and possibly seizures. Usually glucose therapy is given at the start of an attack, with saline if there is hyponatraemia, but it is advisable to give Normosang® (haem arginate) as soon as possible, as this treatment is far more reliable.

Precautions should be taken to avoid the stimuli that can lead to acute attacks, even if the person has never had an attack. This means not drinking alcohol, only taking drugs that are known to be safe, and eating regular meals with a high carbohydrate content. This is particularly important for women, as the changes during the menstrual cycle can provoke attacks. The wearing of a MedicAlert bracelet is advisable for patients who have acute attacks, to ensure that in an emergency all medical staff are aware of the individual's condition. A printable safe drugs list is available from the Welsh Medicines Agency, via a link on the British Porphyria Association website (www.porphyria.org.uk). This is updated regularly.

Reviewed by Mr and Mrs J Chamberlayne

Adenosine deaminase deficiency

Other names for this condition

- ADA deficiency
- Adenosine aminohydrolase deficiency
- Severe combined immunodeficiency due to adenosine deaminase deficiency

Adenosine deaminase deficiency is a complex disorder with variable phenotypes. In this condition there is a deficiency or an absence of the enzyme adenosine deaminase. In some cases there may be a partial deficiency of the enzyme. Adenosine deaminase is responsible for promoting certain reactions in the immune cells, and a deficiency of the enzyme leads to a build-up of chemicals that either destroy these cells or prevent them from working properly. The specialised immune cells are types of white blood cells called B-cells that are formed in the bone marrow, and also T-cells that are formed in the thymus gland. Individuals with adenosine deaminase deficiency lack the body's normal protection against different types of infections.

The disorder is genetically inherited from the parents in an autosomal recessive fashion.

This disorder generally presents within the first 2 years of life. Symptoms that commonly occur include diarrhoea and failure to grow and gain weight (failure to thrive). Affected individuals are highly susceptible to repeated severe infections (viral, fungal, bacterial and protozoal), and may also experience persistent thrush (candidiasis). These infections can be very serious in an individual with this disorder, and may be life threatening. The severity of the symptoms can vary, as some individuals have a milder form that often presents later in childhood.

The possibility of adenosine deaminase deficiency should be considered in any child with candidiasis, especially when there is evidence of autosomal recessive inheritance. This disorder is diagnosed by measuring the enzyme activity in red blood cells. Prenatal diagnosis is available by chorionic villus sampling and amniocentesis. Treatment of this disorder can involve enzyme replacement therapy using bovine adenosine deaminase (bovine ADA), joined to a chemical called polyethylene glycol (PEG) to form PEG–ADA. It is given in the form of an injection every 1 to 2 weeks, and it restores the immune response. The ultimate treatment is a bone-marrow transplant from a suitable donor. This is usually a sibling who has a matched tissue type, because the immune system is so vulnerable that there can be a higher rate of rejection.

Reviewed by Dr MJ Henderson

Adenylosuccinate lyase deficiency

Other names for this condition
- Adenylosuccinase deficiency
- ADSL deficiency
- Succinylpurinemic autism

Adenylosuccinate lyase deficiency is a rare disorder characterised by a deficiency or an absence of the enzyme adenylosuccinate lyase. This enzyme catalyses two separate steps in the pathways of purine nucleotide synthesis. ADSL deficiency results in a blockage in these pathways and the build-up of two unusual chemical compounds, succinylaminoimidazole carboxamide riboside (SAICAR) and adenylosuccinic acid (AMPS), in the body. Both have a toxic effect on the brain and cause the symptoms of this condition. There are four forms of this disorder.

This disorder is genetically inherited from the parents in an autosomal recessive fashion.

Symptoms of this disorder usually appear during the first 2 years of life, and may include a delay in physical and mental development, epileptic seizures, growth delays, muscle weakness and behavioural difficulties similar to those seen in autism, such as failure to make eye contact, repetitive behaviour and temper tantrums. Other symptoms include low muscle tone (except in the hands and feet, where there is high muscle tone), feeding problems, a squint (strabismus), muscle wasting and twitching of the muscles. The range and severity of symptoms vary from one individual to another. The prognosis for those affected by this disorder is poor. Most people with adenylosuccinate lyase deficiency have the type I disorder, which is characterised by a severe delay in mental development, autistic features, epilepsy and low muscle tone. Many of these individuals die in early infancy. Type II is characterised by hearing difficulties and a delay in mental and visual development. The delay in mental development is less severe than that in Type I. This form has a more positive prognosis, with some individuals reaching their twenties or thirties. Type III is characterised by severe growth problems, severe delays in mental development and muscle wasting. Type IV is a mixture of type I and type II.

Adenylosuccinate lyase deficiency can be diagnosed by newborn screening programmes, and the diagnosis can be confirmed by a urine test. Prenatal diagnosis is available in some cases. Treatment for individuals with this disease aims to provide relief of any symptoms and support in the care of the individual. Anti-epileptic drugs may be used to treat seizures. Genetic counselling may be of benefit to individuals affected by this disorder.

Reviewed by Dr A Simmonds

Dihydropyrimidine dehydrogenase deficiency

Other names for this condition
- Combined uraciluria–thyminuria

In this disorder there is a deficiency or an absence of an enzyme called dihydropyrimidine dehydrogenase. This enzyme is required to break down uracil into dihydrouracil, and to break down thymine into dihydrothymine. The enzyme deficiency leads to a build-up of uracil and dihydrouracil, which causes the symptoms of the condition. Uracil and thymine are important for the function of DNA. There are two forms of this condition:

- an infantile form in which symptoms appear in early infancy
- a later-onset form in which symptoms present later in life.

This disorder is genetically inherited from the parents in an autosomal recessive fashion.

In the infantile form, symptoms may include seizures, a delay in physical and mental development, including growth and speech development, an increase in the tone of the muscles, causing muscle rigidity and tension (hypertonia), heightened reflex responses (hyperreflexia) and a small-sized head (microcephaly). The severity and range of symptoms vary form one individual to another. Those with a complete absence of the enzyme may have a large number of the above symptoms, whereas individuals with a milder deficiency may present with seizures alone.

The later-onset form is also known as the pharmacogenic form. This is because symptoms occur following exposure to 5-fluorouracil, which is a chemotherapeutic agent used in the treatment of some cancers. This can lead to a range of symptoms, including severe diarrhoea, swelling, irritation, and ulceration of the mucosal cells that line the digestive tract (mucositis), a deficiency of one or more of the different types of blood cells (cytopenia), an inability to coordinate muscle movements (ataxia), and muscle weakness. In this form of the disorder, the deficiency of dihydropyrimidine dehydrogenase is only partial.

Treatment for individuals with the early-onset form of the disorder aims to relieve any symptoms and provide support in the care of the individual. Symptoms are commonly non-progressive, so usually remain the same. However, a few deaths have been documented in children who have been severely affected. In the adult-onset form, cancer symptoms have slowly resolved after the discontinuation of chemotherapeutic agents containing 5-fluorouracil.

Reviewed by Dr G Besley

Lesch–Nyhan disease

Other names for this condition
- Hereditary hyperuricaemia and choreoathetosis syndrome
- HGPRT, absence of
- HPRT, absence of
- Hyperuricaemia, choreoathetosis, self-mutilation syndrome
- Hyperuricaemia–oligophrenia
- Hypoxanthine–guanine phosphoribosyltranferase deficiency (complete absence of HPRT)
- Juvenile gout, choreoathetosis, and mental retardation syndrome
- Lesch–Nyhan syndrome

This disorder belongs to a group of conditions known as purine metabolic disorders. It is a rare and devastating genetic disorder associated with an almost complete absence of the enzyme hypoxanthine–guanine phosphoribosyltransferase (HGPRT), which metabolises hypoxanthine and guanine to uric acid, the nucleotides IMP and GMP. The disorder is characterised by increased levels of uric acid in the blood and urine and by the absence of the enzyme HPRT.

This disorder may occur spontaneously, but is usually inherited by a method called X-linked inheritance.

Symptoms usually begin to appear between the ages of 3 and 6 months. Often the first symptom is the presence of orange crystal-like deposits in the nappies of affected infants. The deposits are uric acid (also known as urate) crystals, and are caused by increased levels of uric acid in the urine. High uric acid levels in the circulation may also cause sodium urate crystals to form in the joints, kidneys, central nervous system and other tissues of the body. Other symptoms include kidney stones, impaired kidney function, renal disease and blood in the urine. Individuals with this disorder are irritable and display uncontrolled aggression.

Symptoms may include purposeless repetitive movements such as shoulder raising and facial grimacing, destructive chewing of fingertips or lips, compulsive self-injury, head banging, leg banging, rubbing the body until it is raw, and kicking and head butting others, followed by repeated apologies for this behaviour. Behaviour problems may escalate as the child gets older. Self-injury may be related to abnormalities in the metabolism of the neurotransmitters serotonin or dopamine. Those affected by this disorder may have difficulty in swallowing (dysphagia) and eating, delayed motor development followed by unusual movements and increased deep tendon reflexes, gout-like swelling of the joints, movement disorder, speech impairment, exaggerated reflexes (hyperreflexia), vomiting, and a combination of slow writhing involuntary movements and fast jerky movements (choreoathetoid movements). Severe and progressive disability is likely.

No treatment exists for this condition. Haloperidol has been tried, and although it decreases the uric acid levels, it does not improve the neurological outcome. Some symptoms may be relieved by giving carbidopa/levodopa, diazepam, phenobarbital or haloperidol. The patient's teeth may have been removed in the past to limit self-destructive behaviour, but the use of mouth-guards should be tried first. Treatment for individuals with this disease aims to relieve any symptoms and to provide support in the care of the individual. Affected individuals become fearful and upset when left unrestrained or unprotected. In the past the outcome was likely to be poor, but it has been improved by the encouragement of dedicated parents. Genetic counselling may be of benefit to the families of individuals affected by this disorder.

Reviewed by Dr A Simmonds

Myoadenylate deaminase deficiency

Other names for this condition

- MAD deficiency

Myoadenylate deaminase deficiency is a rare metabolic disorder that is characterised by a deficiency of the muscle enzyme adenosine monophosphate (AMP) deaminase enzyme. AMP deaminase and the purine nucleotide cycle have an important role in providing energy for skeletal muscles during exercise. There are two forms of myoadenylate deaminase deficiency, namely an acquired form and an inherited form. This summary will focus on the inherited form.

This disorder is genetically inherited from the parents in an autosomal recessive fashion.

Symptoms of this disorder can present at any time after the age of 2 years, and mainly occur after moderate to vigorous exercise. They include tiring easily, muscle cramps and muscle pain. There may also be an increase in blood serum levels of the muscle enzyme creatine kinase, due to muscle damage. In this disorder the skeletal muscle fails to produce ammonia during exercise. This mild disorder only affects skeletal muscle.

The disorder can be diagnosed by testing whether the skeletal muscle fails to produce ammonia during exercise. A muscle biopsy and blood tests may also be necessary. Treatment of the disorder aims to relieve any symptoms and to provide support in the care of the individual. Administration of ribose may be of benefit, but is only effective for short periods of time. It increases stamina and may eliminate symptoms in some individuals, but may be ineffective in others.

Reviewed by Dr L Fairbanks

Purine nucleoside phosphorylase deficiency

Other names for this condition

- PNP deficiency

Purine nucleoside phosphorylase deficiency is a rare disorder of purine metabolism in which the normal breakdown (catabolism) of the nucleosides inosine and guanosine to their constituent purine bases – hypoxanthine and guanine – does not occur. Purine nucleosides are derived from nucleotides such as ATP and the nucleic acids that make up our DNA, and they contain a sugar (ribose) and a purine base. When this breakdown is interrupted, there is a build-up of the corresponding nucleosides coupled with the excretion of reduced amounts of the constituent purine bases and uric acid.

This disorder is inherited from the parents in an autosomal recessive manner.

Symptoms of the disorder generally become apparent around the age of 2 to 3 years, but sometimes appear up to the age of 7 years. The main symptom is recurrent infections. Affected individuals are particularly prone to viral infections, including chickenpox and mumps. Other symptoms include a low red blood cell count (anaemia), shaky movements and unsteady gait (ataxia), tremor and severe immune deficiency.

This disorder can be diagnosed by urine tests that demonstrate decreased levels of uric acid, and by enzyme tests on red blood cells, providing that there have been no prior blood transfusions. Treatment includes bone-marrow transplantation and irradiated blood transfusions. All other treatments aim to prevent infections, relieve any symptoms and provide support in the care of the individual.

Reviewed by Dr A Simmonds

Pyrimidine 5′-nucleotidase deficiency

Other names for this condition

- UMP hydrolase deficiency

This is a rare disorder caused by a deficiency of the enzyme pyrimidine 5′-nucleotidase (also known as UMP hydrolase). This enzyme removes phosphate groups from organic compounds known as pyrimidine-5′-ribomonophosphates, converting the latter to the corresponding compounds that consist of a nitrogen-containing pyrimidine base and a sugar (nucleoside).

This disorder is inherited from the parents in an autosomal recessive manner.

The symptoms of pyrimidine 5′-nucleotidase deficiency may present at any age. The main symptom is non-spherocytic haemolytic anaemia, characterised by basophilic stippling. Other findings may include an enlarged spleen (splenomegaly), enlarged kidneys, gallstones, and the excretion of iron in the urine. There may be an increase in the number of immature red blood cells (reticulocytosis), and red blood cells may be unequal in size (anisocytosis). Additional findings include an increase in the yellowish pigment found in bile (bilirubin), and increased levels of glutathione in the red blood cells.

This disorder should be suspected in any individual who has mild chronic non-spherocytic haemolytic anaemia with basophilic stippling. It can be diagnosed by enzyme analysis and by demonstrating the accumulation of pyrimidine nucleotides in red blood cells. Pyrimidine 5′-nucleotidase deficiency is a relatively harmless disorder. If the anaemia becomes severe, a transfusion may be necessary. However, this is rarely needed.

Reviewed by Dr L Fairbanks

Variegate porphyria

Other names for this condition
- VP
- South African porphyria

This disorder belongs to a group of conditions known as the porphyrias. In this form of porphyria there is a deficiency of the enzyme protoporphyrinogen oxidase, which slows down the conversion of aminolevulinic acid (ALA) into haem. This leads to a build-up of porphyrins and causes skin sensitivity upon exposure to light. Unfortunately, there is also a feedback mechanism that leads to a build-up of aminolevulinic acid (ALA), and of porphobilinogen (PBG) produced directly from ALA, which can cause acute attacks that affect the nervous system.

This disorder is inherited in an autosomal dominant manner. Variegate porphyria is most common in individuals of white South African descent, and is less frequent in other populations.

Affected individuals usually develop symptoms after they have reached puberty. However, about four out of five individuals who inherit the gene for this condition do not display any symptoms at all. Those who do show symptoms may have obvious skin problems, or acute attacks, or both. Acute attacks are often provoked by certain drugs, alcohol, hormonal changes or a diet low in carbohydrate. Anyone with variegate porphyria should carry a list of safe drugs, and should also make sure that any doctor treating them has such a list.

The main symptom of an acute attack is abdominal pain (or sometimes back pain) and this may be accompanied by nausea, vomiting, constipation, confusion and hallucinations. The urine can be red or brownish (particularly if left to stand for testing) due to an excess of porphyrins. The salt content of the blood may fall (hyponatraemia), and a blood test is needed to check whether this needs to be treated. There may also be pain in the arms and legs, a rapid heartbeat, increased blood pressure, muscle weakness and possibly seizures. Usually glucose therapy is given at the start of an attack, with saline if there is hyponatraemia, but it is advisable to give Normosang (haem arginate) as soon as possible, as this treatment is far more reliable.

Precautions should be taken to avoid the stimuli that can lead to acute attacks, even if the person has never had an attack. This means not drinking alcohol, only taking drugs that are known to be safe, and eating regular meals that have a high carbohydrate content. This is particularly important for women, as the changes that occur during the menstrual cycle can provoke attacks. The wearing of a MedicAlert bracelet is advisable for patients who have acute attacks, to ensure that in an emergency all medical staff are aware of the individual's condition. A printable safe drugs list is available from the Welsh Medicines Agency, via a link on the British Porphyria Association website (www.porphyria.org.uk). This is updated regularly.

Sensitivity to sunlight, which can cause the skin to burn and blister, seems to vary and can be independent of attacks. Scarring may occur if the skin is not protected against the sun. Exposure to direct sunlight should be avoided. However, if this is impossible, the wearing of a hat, long sleeves and long trousers or a long skirt is recommended. Sunscreens with a high UVA factor (look on the back of the bottle) are recommended, although some individuals may find that sunblock is needed.

Reviewed by Mr and Mrs J Chamberlayne

Xanthine oxidase deficiency

Other names for this condition
- Hereditary xanthinuria
- Xanthine dehydrogenase deficiency
- XDH deficiency

Xanthine oxidase deficiency is a genetic disorder caused by a deficiency of the enzyme xanthine dehydrogenase. This enzyme is needed to convert xanthine to uric acid during the breakdown of purine. In this disorder there is a build-up of xanthine because it cannot be converted to uric acid. Xanthine oxidase deficiency may be combined with *sulphite oxidase deficiency* and *aldehyde oxidase deficiency*, resulting in the combined *molybdenum cofactor deficiency*.

Both xanthine oxidase and the combined disorder are inherited in an autosomal recessive fashion.

Symptoms of xanthine oxidase deficiency may include irritability, blood in the urine (haematuria), colic, and crystal-like deposits in the urine. Symptoms commonly present following diarrhoea, infection or exercise. This disorder can lead to muscle disease caused by xanthine deposits in the muscle, as well as renal disease, kidney stones and urinary tract problems due to the presence of xanthine stones. The combined disorder can result in more severe symptoms, including feeding difficulties and seizures shortly after birth, jerky movements, increased muscle tone (hypertonia) or decreased muscle tone (hypotonia), dislocation of the lens of the eye, and severe developmental delay and learning difficulties.

This disorder is diagnosed by blood and urine tests, and is demonstrated by a low level of uric acid, which is replaced by xanthine in the blood and urine. Treatment for this disorder involves avoiding food and drinks that have a high purine content. It is important that affected individuals drink plenty of fluids and avoid becoming dehydrated.

Reviewed by Dr L Fairbanks

Chapter 7

Hormone disorders

Hormone disorders are caused by a defect in the production of hormones by the appropriate glands. Hormones are secreted into the bloodstream so that they can access all of the cells in the body. The symptoms of the different hormone disorders depend on which gland or hormone is not functioning correctly.

- The adrenal glands are located above each of the kidneys. Their role is to secrete adrenaline, aldosterone and cortisol to help to control kidney function and body fluid concentrations, and to maintain blood pressure and salt levels in the body. In cases of overproduction, they also produce sex hormones.
- The neuroendocrine glands are located in the pancreas. Their role is to secrete insulin and somatostatin to help to control salt and blood sugar levels.
- The parathyroid gland is located behind the thyroid gland. It secretes parathyroid hormone and controls the body's calcium levels. In some cases it produces too much (hyperparathyroidism) or, more rarely, too little (hypoparathyroidism) parathyroid hormone, in both cases causing calcium imbalances and other serious complications.
- The pituitary gland is located at the base of the brain. It secretes adrenocortico-trophic hormone (ACTH, also known as corticotrophin), antidiuretic hormone (ADH), growth hormone, prolactin, thyroid-stimulating hormone and the gona-dotrophins, namely luteinising hormone (LH) and follicle-stimulating hormone (FSH).
- The thyroid gland is located at the front of the neck. It secretes thyroid hormone and controls the body's metabolism by increasing cellular activity in nearly all of the body's tissues.

Pseudohypoaldosteronism type 1

Other names for this condition

- PHA1
- Pseudohypoaldosteronism type 1 – autosomal dominant form
- Pseudohypoaldosteronism type 1 – autosomal recessive form

Pseudohypoaldosteronism type 1 is a rare disorder characterised by salt wasting in infancy, and caused by certain organs being unresponsive to mineralocorticoids. The latter are steroid hormones that are necessary for the regulation of salt and water balance. Salt wasting occurs when the kidneys excrete large amounts of salt even though the body appears to need it.

There are two forms of this disorder:

- pseudohypoaldosteronism type 1 – autosomal dominant form. This is caused by defects in the mineralocorticoid receptor gene, which is located on the long arm of chromosome 4
- pseudohypoaldosteronism type 1 – autosomal recessive form. This is caused by defects in genes on either the short arm of chromosome 16 or the short arm of chromosome 12.

In the autosomal dominant form of pseudohypoaldosteronism type 1, the symptoms are more severe and persist into adulthood, whereas in the autosomal recessive form the symptoms may be severe at birth, but they will become milder with age. In this form, the mineralocorticoid resistance mainly occurs in the kidney, the salivary glands, sweat and the tissue covering the main part of the large intestine (colonic epithelium). In the autosomal dominant form, the resistance is limited to the kidney. Symptoms include dehydration, failure to grow or gain weight (failure to thrive), refusal to feed, recurring respiratory infections, low blood pressure, short stature, vomiting, a low concentration of sodium in the blood (hyponatraemia), and an abnormally high concentration of potassium in the blood (hyperkalaemia), due to failure of the kidneys to excrete it.

Pseudohypoaldosteronism type 1 is diagnosed by clinical testing. Treatment of this condition involves giving high doses of salt and the administration of drugs such as carbenoxolone, dexamethasone and fludrocortisone.

Reviewed by Dr R Stanhope

ACTH deficiency

Other names for this condition

- Adrenocorticotrophic hormone deficiency, isolated

In this disorder, there is a deficiency or an absence of adrenocorticotrophic hormone (ACTH), which is produced by the pituitary gland in the brain. ACTH stimulates the production of another hormone, known as cortisol, which is found in the adrenal glands. The adrenal glands are located above each kidney. The loss of cortisol in ACTH deficiency can lead to serious problems. This disorder can also affect other hormones. Isolated ACTH deficiency is incredibly rare, and it is much more common for ACTH deficiency to be a feature of hypopituitarism.

The cause of most cases of ACTH deficiency is not yet known. It has been suggested that a defect in the brain structure or in the pituitary gland may result in this disorder.

There is a congenital form (present at birth) of ACTH deficiency, which is believed to be caused by a defect in genes located on chromosomes 1 and 8. This form of the disorder is inherited from the parents in an autosomal recessive fashion.

Symptoms of this condition usually first appear during adulthood. However, a few cases of symptoms occurring in childhood have been reported. Symptoms commonly include weight loss, lack of appetite, muscle weakness, nausea, vomiting, low blood sugar levels (hypoglycaemia), low levels of sodium in the blood (hyponatraemia), high levels of potassium in the blood (hyperkalaemia), and low blood pressure (hypotension).

Some adrenal hormones are affected, which may include androgens (precursors of the male sex hormones). Female individuals may have reduced amounts of pubic and underarm hair, and may experience nausea and have pale skin. Depression and other psychiatric problems may occur in individuals with this disorder.

ACTH deficiency is diagnosed on the basis of blood tests and occasionally insulin tolerance tests. It is strongly recommended that tests for other hormone deficiencies be conducted. Treatment of this disorder involves hormone replacement therapy, by replacing the cortisol whose production would normally be stimulated by ACTH. Hydrocortisone or cortisone may be given in divided doses to correct the hormone deficiency. These treatments will correct the deficiency or absence of ACTH, relieve the symptoms and allow the affected individual to lead a normal life. Increased doses of cortisone may be required in the presence of moderate or severe stress.

Reviewed by Professor J Wass

Albright hereditary osteodystrophy

Other names for this condition

- AHO
- Albright's IV
- Albright's syndrome
- Fuller–Albright syndrome 1
- Pseudohypoparathyroidism
- PHP
- PHPT
- Pseudo-pseudohypoparathyroidism
- PPHP

Albright hereditary osteodystrophy is a rare disorder that can lead to the appearance of certain physical characteristics, including a short stature in adulthood, a tendency to have weight problems, and shortening of some of the bones in the hands and feet. The characteristics of this disorder are associated with a resistance to parathyroid hormone (pseudohypoparathyroidism type 1a) and to other hormones.

There are two forms of Albright hereditary osteodystrophy (AHO):

- AHO with pseudohypoparathyroidism
- AHO with pseudo-pseudohypoparathyroidism.

Both have the same cause, and both forms can occur within the same family.

This disorder is inherited in an autosomal dominant manner.

The main effects of Albright hereditary osteodystrophy are subtle physical changes. On reaching adulthood, affected individuals tend to be short in stature. Symptoms include characteristic facial features, such as a rounded face, a flattened nose, colour abnormalities in the retina, cataracts, a thickened skull and a short neck. Some individuals may have dental abnormalities, such as problems relating to the enamel, missing teeth due to their failure to develop (anodontia) or the late eruption of teeth. It is not known why this is so, but sufferers are prone to being overweight. Sometimes this may be related to a malfunctioning thyroid gland, but not in all cases.

Other symptoms that can present in this disease include a delay in learning skills such as speaking and walking. Walking may be difficult due to the legs being curved inwards (genu valgum), foot abnormalities, hip problems and lower limb deficiency. Affected individuals may have muscular weakness (hemiparesis) or paralysis (hemiplegia) of one side of the body, or over-reactive reflexes and some shortening of some of the bones in the hands and feet. Individuals with AHO commonly have small hard lumps (subcutaneous ossifications) under the skin. Most of these are small and do not cause any problems. The range and severity of these symptoms can vary from one individual to another.

In addition to the symptoms described above, if an individual has the pseudohypoparathyroidism (PHP) form of AHO there may be other symptoms. In this form of the disorder the body is unable to respond to parathyroid hormone, which maintains the levels of calcium in the blood. Therefore individuals with PHP usually have low calcium levels, which can cause tingling in the fingers, muscle cramps and possible fits (seizures). Sometimes there may also be a decrease in the production of thyroid hormone.

If an individual has the pseudo-pseudohypoparathyroidism (PPHP) form of AHO, they will have some of the features of AHO, but the body responds to parathyroid hormone and they will have normal calcium levels.

Treatment for this disorder includes maintaining a healthy and varied diet to prevent any excessive weight gain. Hypothyroidism must be treated with a replacement thyroid hormone. If a learning disability is involved, extra assistance at school will be of benefit. The pseudohypoparathyroidism form requires treatment with a vitamin D compound, which will encourage the reabsorption of calcium in the kidneys. Calcium supplements and other drugs that reduce the amount of calcium that is excreted by the body may also be of benefit. Eye problems such as cataracts need to be assessed by an ophthalmologist and appropriate treatment given.

Reviewed by Professor PM Stewart

Bannayan–Riley–Ruvalcaba syndrome

Other names for this condition

- Bannayan syndrome
- Bannayan–Zonana syndrome
- BRRS
- BZS
- Cowden/Bannayan–Riley–Ruvalcaba overlap syndrome
- Macrocephaly, multiple lipomas and haemangiomata
- Macrocephaly, pseudopapilloedema and multiple haemangiomata
- PTEN hamartoma tumour syndrome
- Riley–Smith syndrome
- RMSS
- Ruvalcaba–Myhre syndrome
- Ruvalcaba–Myhre–Smith syndrome

This disorder is a combination of three conditions, formerly considered to be separate disorders, known as Bannayan–Zonana syndrome, Riley–Smith syndrome and Ruvalcaba–Myhre–Smith syndrome. There is still some debate as to whether these are three separate conditions, or slightly different forms of the same disorder.

Bannayan–Riley–Ruvalcaba syndrome is inherited in an autosomal dominant manner.

An early indication of this disorder is commonly a high birth weight and body length. This fast growth may continue after birth, but slows with age, so that by adulthood affected individuals have a normal stature. Other symptoms that may be present at birth or which can develop during infancy may include a large-sized head (macrocephaly) that is often long and narrow (scaphocephaly), a loss of muscle tone (hypotonia), a delay in physical and mental development, including speech, hyper-extendable joints, curving of the spine (scoliosis), and muscle weakness due to the storage of certain lipids (fats) in the muscles. Males develop dark freckle-like spots on the skin, especially in the genital region, and some individuals have seizures.

Non-cancerous (benign) tumour-like growths, known as hamartomas, commonly develop. These may consist of fatty tissue (lipomas) and/or clusters of blood vessels (haemangiomas) and/or widened lymph vessels (lymphangiomas). They occur beneath the surface of the skin, and they vary in size and number. Some individuals have small growths known as polyps in the intestines and occasionally at the back of the throat. In addition, there may be changes to the eyes, such as squints (strabismus), widely spaced eyes (ocular hypertelorism), abnormal elevation of the optic disc at the back of the eye (pseudopapilloedema) and visual impairment (amblyopia). It should be noted that the range and severity of symptoms vary from one individual to another.

Treatment of this condition aims to relieve the symptoms. Eye specialists (ophthalmologists) should be consulted to determine whether the eyes are affected. Physical and speech therapy can be of benefit, as can educational support at school. Sometimes the tumour-like growths (hamartomas) cause complications and may need to be removed. Individuals with this condition may be more prone to developing other tumours and malignancies, and should therefore be more closely monitored to ensure that these are detected early.

Reviewed by Dr K Lachlan

Coffin–Siris syndrome

Other names for this condition
- Dwarfism–onychodysplasia
- Fifth-digit syndrome
- Mental retardation with hypoplastic fifth fingernails and toenails
- Short stature–onychodysplasia

Coffin–Siris syndrome is a rare genetic disorder in which severe learning disability and short stature are associated with sparse scalp hair but excess hair elsewhere, especially on the face, where the eyebrows may be conjoined, but also over the back. Facial features tend to include thick lips, a flat nasal bridge and a large mouth. There is characteristically underdevelopment of the nails, especially that of the fifth finger and the toenails, but the whole digit may be shortened. Joint laxity and loss of muscle tone (hypotonia) have often been noted.

The disorder can affect both sexes, and is said to be inherited in an autosomal recessive manner, but there have been a few cases in which a variety of chromosome abnormalities have been identified.

Symptoms of this disorder appear early in life and may include vomiting, delayed growth, loss of muscle tone (hypotonia), frequent infections, abnormally loose joints, delayed bone age and other skeletal abnormalities. The latter can include spinal/vertebral malformations, hip deformations (coxa valga), a dislocated elbow, and abnormally small or absent knee caps. Breathing difficulties may be a result of a blockage caused by a bony layer of tissue (choanal atresia).

Apart from the characteristic features described above, other symptoms and signs of the disorder may include a small head (microcephaly), drooping of the eyelids (ptosis), a hernia, undescended testes, heart abnormalities, dislocation of the inner forearm bone at the elbow, and a partial or complete absence of the nerve fibres that connect the two hemispheres of the brain (agenesis of corpus callosum). A brain abnormality known as Dandy–Walker syndrome may also be present.

Coffin–Siris syndrome is diagnosed on the basis of the characteristic clinical features and the exclusion of other disorders that can mimic the condition, such as biotinidase deficiency. There are no specific tests to confirm the clinical diagnosis, as no specific gene for the condition has yet been identified. There is no specific treatment other than the treatment of any complications that may be present and assisting the child with their learning disability. Genetic counselling may be of benefit to individuals affected by this disorder.

Reviewed by Dr A Fryer

Congenital adrenal hyperplasia – 3-beta-hydroxysteroid dehydrogenase

---

Other names for this condition
- 3β-HSD

Congenital adrenal hyperplasia (CAH) refers to a group of disorders in which the functioning of the adrenal glands is impaired. The adrenal glands are located above each of the kidneys. They produce three essential steroid hormones, namely cortisol (stress hormone), aldosterone (salt-retaining hormone) and androgens (a group of male sex hormones). The production of these hormones is stimulated by the pituitary gland, which is located in the brain.

In this form of CAH there is a deficiency of the enzyme 3-beta-hydroxysteroid dehydrogenase. This leads to a reduction in the amount of cortisol, aldosterone and androgen produced by the adrenal glands. When insufficient cortisol is produced, the pituitary gland keeps signalling to the adrenal glands to make more by sending an adrenal-stimulating hormone. If the levels of the adrenal-stimulating hormone remain elevated over a prolonged period, the adrenal glands increase in size (hyperplasia).

This disorder is inherited from the parents in an autosomal recessive manner. This form of CAH accounts for 3% of all cases of CAH, and has an incidence of 1 in 500,000.

Symptoms commonly present in newborns with ambiguous genitalia. Girls often present with an enlarged clitoris and fused labia, whereas boys can have undescended testes and hypospadia, where the opening of the uretha is on the underside of the penis. In addition, 'adrenal crises' occur due to stress or illness. These episodes are characterised by dehydration, low blood pressure, vomiting, low levels of salt and sugar in the blood and raised potassium levels. They require prompt treatment with steroid hormones, otherwise unconsciousness and death can occur. This form of CAH can be either mild or severe, and may be detected in early infancy, in adolescence or not until adulthood. In childhood, very early development of secondary sexual characteristics, such as changes in body shape, acne and the development of pubic hair, may occur. Affected individuals may also grow too fast and too early in childhood, and consequently they stop growing too soon, resulting in a shortened adult stature.

Treatment of this disorder includes correcting the lack of cortisol by replacing it with hydrocortisone, prednisolone or dexamethasone. As a result, normal development and onset of puberty should occur. Medical intervention is often required for puberty. The lack of aldosterone in individuals who are classed as 'salt losers' must be corrected by replacing it with fludrocortisone to maintain the salt and water balance in the body. The replacement of these steroid hormones must be continued daily for life. In times of stress and during illness or surgery, extra cortisol replacement is usually needed.

Reviewed by Mrs S Elford

Growth hormone deficiency

Other names for this condition
- GHD

Growth hormone deficiency is a condition in which growth hormone production is reduced or absent during infancy or childhood. Growth hormone is produced by the pituitary gland, which is located at the base of the skull. A deficiency of growth hormone results in a lack of growth in the child. If only growth hormone is deficient, the disorder is known as hypopituitarism. If there is a deficiency of all the homones that are produced by the pituitary gland, the disorder is known as panhypopituitarism.

Growth hormone deficiency can be inherited in an autosomal recessive, an autosomal dominant or an X-linked fashion. In most cases the problem may occur for no apparent reason (in which case it is described as idiopathic). However, in some cases a tumour or a treatment for cancer can disrupt the production of growth hormone.

In most cases this condition is caused by the pituitary gland not developing properly or being damaged in some way so that it is unable to produce sufficient growth hormone to meet the body's needs. Babies with this disorder are usually of normal weight and length at birth. During the newborn period, the infant may have low blood sugar levels. Symptoms of this disorder include an abnormal rate of facial bone development, delayed skeletal development, delayed closure of the front bones of the skull (fontanelles) and a delay in the development of the teeth. Affected individuals may also have fine hair, poor nail growth and a high-pitched voice, and may be obese. Other symptoms may include a small penis in males, and abnormal sexual maturity due to insufficient levels of gonadotrophin which is required for normal sexual development, and which is also produced by the pituitary gland.

The condition is usually confirmed after concerns have been expressed about the child's growth pattern. Specialised testing will be needed to determine whether the individual has growth hormone deficiency, to confirm the diagnosis. Treatment of this disorder includes recombinant human growth hormone injections. The dosage is increased as the child gets bigger, and is usually assessed at approximately 17 years of age to establish whether the treatment needs to be continued into adulthood. Individuals who receive this form of treatment may notice an increase in appetite and a loss of body fat. Those who are given an early diagnosis and who show a good response to treatment are able to reach normal adult height. Genetic counselling may be of benefit to individuals affected by this disorder.

Reviewed by Professor J Wass and the Child Growth Foundation

Hypopituitarism

Other names for this condition

- Pituitary insufficiency

Hypopituitarism is a term used to describe an underactive pituitary gland. It is caused by damage to the front and back part of the gland. The pituitary gland is located at the base of the skull and is attached to the hypothalamus, the part of the brain that controls its function. Because the pituitary gland does not work properly, some of the following hormones may not be produced:

- growth hormone
- thyroid-stimulating hormone (TSH)
- adrenocorticotrophic hormone (ACTH)
- prolactin
- luteinising hormone (LH)
- follicle-stimulating hormone (FSH)
- antidiuretic hormone (ADH).

This disorder may be caused by tumours of the pituitary gland or hypothalamus. It may also be caused by brain tumours, brain surgery, injury to the head, radiation, stroke, or an infection of the brain and its supporting tissues. In some cases, metabolic disorders or immune system diseases may cause hypopituitarism. This disorder may also be a complication following pregnancy (Sheehan's syndrome).

Symptoms of hypopituitarism usually appear slowly, and may vary widely depending on the hormones that are affected. Children with this disorder may experience growth problems and a delay in sexual development. Common symptoms include weakness, tiredness, depression, stress intolerance, low blood sugar levels, loss of appetite, weight loss and abdominal pain. Other symptoms may include dry skin, sensitivity to cold, low blood pressure, headache, confusion, visual problems, hair loss and loss of armpit and/or pubic hair, and growth delay. Affected individuals may also have pale skin, unexplained weight gain, constipation, joint stiffness, muscle weakness, swelling of the face and a hoarse voice. Men may experience loss of facial and body hair, a low libido, impotence, decreased sperm production and abnormal testes, and may be infertile. Women may fail to lactate, may experience vaginal dryness and absent periods, and may be infertile.

This disorder may be diagnosed on the basis of a physical examination, a medical history, a cranial CT and MRI scan, and blood tests to determine which hormones are affected. Treatment may include surgical removal and radiation therapy if the disorder is caused by a pituitary tumour. Hormone replacement therapy is needed, and drugs may also need to be administered to treat infertility. Other treatment aims to relieve any symptoms and to provide support in the care of the individual.

Reviewed by Professor J Wass

Leprechaunism

Other names for this condition

- Donohue syndrome

This disorder is characterised by overdevelopment of the pancreas. The pancreas produces the hormone insulin, which aids the absorption of glucose by cells throughout the body. Abnormal resistance to insulin results in severe hormonal (endocrine) disturbances, which can lead to abnormalities in growth and development.

Leprechaunism is genetically inherited from the parents in an autosomal recessive fashion.

Many of the symptoms that occur in leprechaunism are present at birth (i.e. they are congenital). The common symptoms may include a growth delay (before and after birth), failure to grow or gain weight (failure to thrive), a lack of fatty tissue under the skin (subcutaneous adipose tissue), a delay in the bones becoming fully developed and progressive muscle wasting. Various characteristics can occur as a result of the hormonal imbalance in this disorder. Some of the facial features that may be apparent include large low-set ears, a flat bridge to the nose, large thick lips, a large mouth, widely spaced eyes and a small-sized head (microcephaly). There may also be abnormal darkening and thickening of patches of skin (acanthosis nigricans), the skin may appear to be too large for the body, and other features include excessive hair growth, large hands and feet, and enlargement of the breasts and sexual organs. Occasionally, cysts may develop in the ovaries. The range and severity of the symptoms vary from one individual to another.

Diagnosis may be confirmed on the basis of clinical evaluation, patient history and blood tests. Prenatal diagnosis is available.

The treatment of this disorder is symptomatic and supportive, as it aims to relieve symptoms and make the individual as comfortable as possible. Affected individuals may see specialists with expertise in paediatrics, endocrinology and dermatology. Children with leprechaunism rarely reach primary school age. Genetic counselling is recommended for individuals affected by this disorder.

Reviewed by Dr R Stanhope

Prader–Willi syndrome

Other names for this condition

- Cryptorchidism–dwarfism–subnormal mentality
- H$_3$O
- HHHO
- Hypogenital dystrophy with diabetic tendency
- Hypotonia–hypomentia–hypogonadism–obesity syndrome
- Labhart–Willi syndrome
- Prader–Labhart–Willi–Fancone syndrome
- Prader–Labhart–Willi syndrome
- PWS
- Willi–Prader syndrome

Prader–Willi syndrome is a rare disorder characterised by decreased fetal movement, weak muscle tone (hypotonia), feeding difficulties and failure to grow and gain weight (failure to thrive). This disorder is thought to be caused by a deletion of the Prader–Willi syndrome/Angelman syndrome (PWS/AS) region on the long arm of chromosome 15.

In most cases, Prader–Willi syndrome occurs spontaneously for unknown reasons, although in some cases, according to investigators, the chromosome that is deleted is always paternally derived. When the deletion affects the maternally derived chromosome, it results in a different disorder, known as Angelman syndrome. For further information about the inheritance of this disorder, a genetic counselling service should be consulted.

The symptoms of Prader–Willi syndrome include decreased fetal movement, sleepiness, feeding problems, small hands and feet, genital abnormalities and obesity, especially in the lower body, which is linked with an obsession with eating. Individuals suffering from severe progressive obesity may be at increased risk of developing diabetes or other serious conditions that may lead to potentially life-threatening complications. Those affected by this disorder commonly have strong facial characteristics, including a narrow forehead, a thin upper lip, almond-shaped eyes and unusual crossing of the eyes (strabismus). Curvature of the spine (scoliosis) can cause delays in walking, and children may have learning difficulties, respiratory problems, skin lesions, low temperature and behavioural problems. People affected by this disorder tend to have fair colouring with blue eyes and sun-sensitive skin. They also have a high pain threshold, so if they fall it is not unusual for a broken bone to go undetected. Patients with Prader–Willi syndrome should be monitored for changes in movement and swelling or bruising.

Treatment for individuals with this disorder aims to relieve any symptoms and provide support in the care of the individual. Therapy is needed for behaviour problems, and physiotherapy is used to develop muscle tone and walking. Diet and exercise programmes are needed to control obesity, and those affected require calorie-controlled meals and encouragement to take exercise. Parents need to limit their child's access to food (e.g. by locking cupboards where food is stored and putting food out of reach). A human growth hormone is sometimes used for long-term treatment of growth and weight problems. A tracheotomy or tonsillectomy may help with breathing and sleep problems.

Reviewed by Professor PM Stewart

Chapter 8

Musculoskeletal disorders and connective tissue disorders

Musculoskeletal disorders

The term 'musculoskeletal' refers to the muscles and skeleton. Disorders in this group include those that cause bone deformities, leading to characteristic features such as clubfoot. Some may cause movement problems and susceptibility to fractures due to the bones being brittle. Other disorders may cause the muscles to become weak, so that the affected individual may be unable to carry out day-to-day tasks. In some cases the muscles may waste away.

Connective tissue disorders

Connective tissue joins together and supports structures in the body. There are more than 200 disorders that affect the connective tissues. They are caused by defects in the genes that are responsible for building tissues. These disorders can change the way in which the tissues work and cause abnormalities in the structure and development of certain organs, skin, bones, joints, blood vessels and other structures.

Amyloidosis

The term 'amyloidosis' refers to a group of diseases caused by the accumulation of protein in an abnormal aggregated form that can occur in one or more organs throughout the body. Amyloidosis may occur in conjunction with chronic inflammatory diseases such as rheumatoid arthritis (AA amyloidosis), or as a consequence of a particular bone-marrow disorder (AL amyloidosis). However, amyloidosis can also be inherited, and it is the latter forms that will be covered in this summary.

Other general names that are used for the various inherited forms of amyloidosis

- Familial amyloidotic polyneuropathy (when the disorder mainly affects the nerves)
- Hereditary renal amyloidosis (when it mainly affects the kidneys)
- Hereditary nephropathic amyloidosis (another name for when it mainly affects the kidneys)

The specific forms of hereditary amyloidosis, denoted by the particular abnormal protein responsible, are as follows:

- apolipoprotein AI amyloidosis
- apolipoprotein AII amyloidosis
- cystatin C amyloidosis
- fibrinogen amyloidosis
- gelsolin amyloidosis
- lysozyme amyloidosis
- transthyretin amyloidosis.

Hereditary forms of amyloidosis are inherited in an autosomal dominant fashion.

The different forms of hereditary amyloidosis do vary with regard to the organs of the body that are involved. Sometimes a single organ may be predominantly affected, while in other forms many organs can be affected. For example, hereditary transthyretin amyloidosis mainly affects the nerves, whereas hereditary fibrinogen amyloidosis mainly affects the kidneys. Symptoms therefore vary widely and depend upon which tissues and organs are damaged by the build-up of amyloid protein in each case.

Treatment of inherited amyloidosis aims to relieve any symptoms and provide support in the care of the individual. Kidney failure can be supported by renal dialysis or kidney transplantation, and in some cases liver transplantation can be curative by removing the main source of the genetically abnormal, amyloid-forming protein.

Reviewed by Professor PN Hawkins

Charcot–Marie–Tooth disease

Other names for this condition
- CMT
- Hereditary motor and sensory neuropathy
- HMSN
- Peroneal muscular atrophy

Charcot–Marie–Tooth disease encompasses a group of disorders that affect the nerves which lie outside the brain and spinal cord (the peripheral nerves), and which control many of the muscles in the body. When these nerves are affected, this leads to muscle weakness and the wasting away of tissue, mainly in the legs. 'Charcot–Marie–Tooth' comes from the names of the three doctors (two French, one English) who first described the condition in the 1880s.

There are many forms of this disorder, based on the different gene defects. It is believed that these forms are subdivided into two groups:

- type 1 – demyelinating (where the defect in the protein causes a problem with the myelin sheath surrounding the nerve)
- type 2 – axonal (where the defect lies within the axon of the nerve only).

There is a very rare third type in which the nerves show both demyelination and axonal degeneration. Between 25 and 30 genetic variants have now been discovered, although only four can be tested for in the UK.

It is more common for Charcot–Marie–Tooth disease to be inherited in an autosomal dominant manner. However, there are forms of type 1 and type 2 that are inherited in an autosomal recessive fashion. CMT type 1X is genetically transmitted by X-linked inheritance.

This is a slowly progressing disorder that occurs gradually in adolescence, early adulthood or middle age. The symptoms include muscle weakness in the hands, feet and/or lower legs, problems with motor skills, and low muscle tone (hypotonia) in the lower leg. Reflexes are usually absent. This disorder leads to the gradual loss of the normal use of the feet, hands, legs and arms. Affected individuals may have problems with abnormally hot or cold extremities, and often experience pain (both neuropathic in origin and from walking awkwardly). They may also trip or fall frequently. The feet can be affected, and abnormalities include a high-stepped gait (foot drop), a high foot arch, flat feet and a condition in which the middle joint of a toe bends upwards (hammer toe). In some cases there may be breathing difficulties. This disorder shows wide variation in symptoms and prognosis, and some individuals may not realise that they have the disorder.

Charcot–Marie–Tooth disease can be diagnosed on the basis of a clinical evaluation of symptoms, a detailed family history and a range of specialised tests. Molecular genetic testing is available for some forms of the disorder. There is no effective treatment, but management aims to relieve any symptoms and provide support in the care of the individual. This may include physiotherapy and support for the legs and feet (orthotics). Surgery may be used to correct deformities.

Research into this disorder is ongoing.

Reviewed by the Charcot–Marie–Tooth Support Group, UK

Coffin–Lowry syndrome

Other names for this condition
- CLS

Coffin–Lowry syndrome is a rare genetic disorder characterised by developmental delay, skeletal, facial and digital abnormalities, reduced muscle tone (hypotonia) in infancy, and short stature. It is caused (at least in some cases) by a defect in the *RSK2* gene that encodes a protein that acts as a growth factor regulator. This gene is located on the short arm of the X chromosome in band 22.

This disorder is passed on by X-linked inheritance. This means that the disease is caused by alterations in genes that are carried on the X chromosome. Females have two X chromosomes, and if a faulty or altered gene is carried on one of these chromosomes, there is usually a normal copy on the other X chromosome to partially or completely compensate for the faulty copy. Males, however, have one X and one Y chromosome. If a male carries a faulty gene on his X chromosome, he will develop the disorder because there is only one X chromosome and therefore no normal copy of the gene to compensate for the faulty copy. In Coffin–Lowry syndrome, female carriers often show some manifestations of the condition, which can be very variable in severity. For further information about the inheritance of Coffin–Lowry syndrome, a genetic counselling service should be consulted.

Symptoms are usually more severe in males. Learning difficulties are usually severe in males, whereas in female carriers, IQ falls along a spectrum from normal to severe learning difficulties. The characteristic facial features in males are usually apparent by the second year of life, with a prominent forehead, widely spaced eyes with thickened eyelids with down-slanting folds, a flat bridge to the nose in childhood, and a prominent jaw with prominent lips and chin. The ears appear large and prominent, the facial bones are abnormally thick, and the forehead is square, with a narrowing of the temples. Characteristic changes are seen in the hands, which tend to be large and soft with thick, double-jointed, tapered fingers. Affected individuals may experience feeding and respiratory problems in infancy. Other features that may develop in males include short stature (95% of cases), a pointed or sunken breastbone (80%), curvature of the spine (80%), which can be severe and can affect heart and lung function, and hearing difficulties. A number of other problems occur less commonly, including abnormalities of the mitral valve in the heart, heart muscle involvement, convulsions and sudden 'drop attacks' (which may require treatment), hernias in males and obesity in females. Males with Coffin–Lowry syndrome are usually described as cheerful, easygoing and friendly. A few adult female carriers with psychiatric illnesses have been reported. Life expectancy may be reduced in affected males, but there are no reliable data for this.

The diagnosis of Coffin–Lowry syndrome is usually made on the basis of the clinical features and physical examination. Genetic testing is not usually required for diagnosis, and indeed for a high proportion of patients believed to have CLS, faults have not been identified in the *RSK2* gene. It is possible that *RSK2* may not be the only gene responsible for CLS. On the other hand, there are now a few reports of boys with severe learning disability who have been found to have faults in the *RSK2* gene, but without the other features of CLS. Treatment is mainly dependent on the symptoms. Hearing deficits should be treated early, as should any curvature of the spine. Physiotherapy, speech therapy and educational therapy should be considered. Genetic counselling is recommended for families with an affected child.

Reviewed by Dr A Fryer

Epidermolysis bullosa

Other names for this condition

- EB

Epidermolysis bullosa (EB) is a rare disorder that is characterised by extremely fragile skin that develops painful blisters and open wounds when it is subjected to minimal everyday friction and trauma. Most cases are inherited, but very rarely cases may be acquired (EB aquisita, a bullous disorder characterised by autoimmunity to type VII collagen).

The inherited form of EB has three main subtypes, namely epidermolysis bullosa simplex (EBS), dystrophic epidermolysis bullosa (DEB) and junctional epidermolysis bullosa (JEB). Each form is based on the depth of the skin to which the blisters extend, together with the absence of specific vital proteins that give the skin its strength. In mild forms the blisters may occur only on the hands and feet, but in other forms they may be more widespread.

This disorder can be inherited in either an autosomal recessive or an autosomal dominant manner.

The symptoms of epidermolysis bullosa vary depending on the form of the disorder. In the simplex form, blisters occur on the outer layers of the skin. This form can be divided into two subtypes, namely the Weber–Cockayne variant and the Dowling–Meara variant. In the Weber–Cockayne variant the blisters are usually found on the feet and hands. The Dowling–Meara variant presents shortly after birth or later, and the blisters occur over much of the body. Individuals affected by this variant may also have growth problems resulting from difficulties with feeding due to blisters in the mouth and severe gastro-oesophageal reflux. Later complications include thickened hard skin over the palms and soles (hyperatosis).

In junctional epidermolysis bullosa (JEB), blisters occur on the deeper layers of skin. There are three main subtypes of this form, namely the Herlitz variant, the non-Herlitz variant and junctional EB with pyloric atresia. Herlitz JEB has a very poor prognosis, with few infants surviving beyond 1 year of age. Death results from a combination of failure to thrive, breathing difficulties and sepsis. Non-Herlitz JEB has a better prognosis. Some individuals affected by this variant have very few skin problems, while others suffer from chronic ulceration, typically on the shins. Hair loss is common in those with non-Herlitz JEB. Junctional EB with pyloric atresia is associated with a blockage to the outlet of the stomach, which requires corrective surgery. This type of EB also carries a very poor prognosis, with a high percentage of those affected dying in early infancy. In all types of JEB, those affected have abnormal dental enamel, and the survivors require extensive dental restoration.

The dystrophic form of epidermolysis bullosa is either present at birth or occurs shortly afterwards. This form can be subdivided into a dominant variant and a recessive variant, in which there is wide variation in severity. Individuals with the dominant and mild recessive variants can lead a fairly normal life, with blistering and wounds limited to sites of trauma, such as knees, ankles and elbows. Those severely affected by the recessive variant have widespread blisters and wounds over most of the body. Internal blistering occurs in the mouth and oesophagus. Blisters on the cornea of the eye are common, and repeated blistering can result in reduced vision. There is a tendency for blistering to heal with a contractual scar, leading to progressive loss of mobility and reduced function in the hands as a result of fusion of the fingers. Internal scarring leads to feeding and swallowing difficulties, and operations to dilate strictures in the oesophagus are required. In severe cases, feeding directly into the stomach using a gastrostomy tube is necessary to maintain good nutrition. In adulthood, those who are severely affected have a high likelihood of developing aggressive skin cancer in the form of squamous-cell carcinoma, which in many cases can be fatal.

Epidermolysis bullosa can be diagnosed on the basis of a physical examination and medical family history in cases of known dominant inheritance. Skin biopsy and analysis of DNA from blood samples are required in individuals with no family history of EB. Prenatal diagnosis is available for severe types of EB following the birth of an affected infant. Treatment of this disorder is based on relieving symptoms and providing support for the individual. Those who are severely affected benefit from multi-disciplinary care within a specialised centre. A cool environment should be maintained. Antibiotics may be given for any infections that may occur. A high-protein diet can prevent malnutrition, and diets should be monitored, especially in the case of individuals with a severe form of EB. Iron supplements may be given for severe anaemia, or blood transfusions may be required. Regular dental care is needed. Blisters and wounds need specialised dressings that can be removed atraumatically.

Reviewed by Ms J Denyer

Hutchinson–Gilford progeria

Other names for this condition
- HGPS
- Hutchinson–Gilford progeria syndrome
- Hutchinson–Gilford syndrome
- Premature ageing syndrome
- Progeria
- Progeria of childhood

Hutchinson–Gilford progeria is a very rare genetic disorder characterised by rapid premature ageing in children. It is caused by a defect in the *LMNA* gene that codes for the lamin A protein. This protein is needed to hold the nucleus of a cell together. It is believed that the premature ageing occurs because the cell nucleus becomes unstable. There are several different forms of progeria, but Hutchinson–Gilford progeria is the classic type.

Most cases have been found to be due to new autosomal dominant mutations in the *LMNA* gene. However, there are reports that progeria can also be inherited in an autosomal recessive fashion.

This disorder usually presents between 9 and 24 months of age. Symptoms that may be apparent at birth (congenital symptoms) include dry shiny hard skin over the lower half of the body, and certain characteristic facial features, including bluish discoloration and nose abnormalities. Symptoms that appear later include severe growth delay and low weight for the height of the individual, underdevelopment of the facial bones (causing a small jaw, a small face and prominent forehead), prominent eyes, thin lips and prominent ears with missing ear lobes. Hair loss may be apparent, and eyebrows and eyelashes may disappear with age. Dental abnormalities may also be present. Individuals with this disorder lose the layer of fat beneath the skin, and may have skeletal abnormalities that include loss of bone density (osteoporosis), degenerative changes that affect many bones in the body, hip deformities, and abnormal tissue forming around some joints, causing joint stiffness and mobility problems. Affected individuals may have an awkward stance and a characteristic walk.

Other bone abnormalities include skull malformations, a short collarbone, thin ribs, a narrow chest, narrow shoulders, a prominent abdomen, and arms and legs that are fragile and susceptible to fractures. Heart problems may be apparent and can also be life threatening in childhood. These problems include an enlarged heart, heart murmurs, thickening of the artery walls resulting in chest pain (angina), obstructed blood flow to the brain, heart failure and heart attack. Other symptoms include prominent veins, brown-coloured skin blotches, brittle yellow nails, a high-pitched voice, hearing difficulties, absent breasts or nipples, and a delay in or absence of sexual maturation.

This disorder can be diagnosed on the basis of a clinical evaluation, physical examination and a range of specialised tests, including the detection of a mutation in the lamin A gene. Treatment of Hutchinson–Gilford progeria aims to relieve any symptoms and provide support in the care of the individual. Research into the use of drugs that could possibly overcome the abnormality in lamin A is ongoing. At present, the prognosis for those affected by this disorder is poor. The average life expectancy of individuals with Hutchinson–Gilford progeria is 13 years, although there is wide variation.

Reviewed by Dr A Fryer

Lafora body disease

Other names for this condition

- EPM2
- Lafora disease
- LBD
- LD
- MELF
- Myoclonic epilepsy of Lafora
- Progressive myoclonic epilepsy type 2

Lafora body disease belongs to a group of disorders known as the progressive myoclonic epilepsies (PMEs), which are characterised by sudden electric-shock-like movements (myoclonus), epileptic fits, and difficulties with walking and speech. These disorders tend to get worse over time. Lafora body disease is one of at least three recognised types of PME, and is characterised by the presence of carbohydrate particles known as Lafora bodies in the cells of the nervous system, muscles and/or skin.

This disorder is genetically inherited from the parents in an autosomal recessive fashion.

Lafora body disease usually presents in late childhood and adolescence. The most common feature is a single seizure in the second decade of life. Symptoms include seizures (which become more frequent with time), myoclonus, incoordination, rapid and severe intellectual decline, and sometimes blindness. This disorder is progressive, and symptoms usually get worse over time. Affected individuals usually die within 10 years of the onset of disease. Rare forms of this disorder have been recorded which present later in life and follow a more benign course.

Treatment for Lafora body disease focuses on medication that provides symptomatic relief, and support in the care of the individual. Clonazepam is sometimes used to treat the myoclonus. Occasionally a combination of medications is required in order to control some of the symptoms.

Reviewed by Dr RA Barker

Lowe syndrome

Other names for this condition
- Cerebro-oculorenal dystrophy
- Lowe–Bickel syndrome
- Lowe–Terry–Maclachlan syndrome
- LS
- OCRL syndrome
- Oculocerebrorenal syndrome
- Oculocerebrorenal syndrome of Lowe
- Renal-oculocerebrodystrophy

Lowe syndrome is a rare metabolic disease that affects males only. However, females can be carriers of the disorder. This disorder is characterised by eye and bone abnormalities, lack of muscle tone (hypotonia) and multiple kidney problems. Lowe syndrome is caused by a mutation in the *OCRL1* gene, which is located on the long arm of the X chromosome. This gene controls production of an enzyme called phosphatidylinositol 4,5-bisphosphate-5-phosphatase. Lack of this enzyme may cause the symptoms that are characteristic of this disorder.

Lowe syndrome is inherited by a method called X-linked inheritance.

Symptoms of this disorder include squinting and flickering of the eye, protrusion of the eyeball from the socket (enophthalmos), caused by the accumulation of water behind the eyeball, and a loss of vision due to excess pressure on the eye (glaucoma). Clouding of the lens of the eye is also common in females, even though they do not have the disorder. Failure to gain weight or increase in height results in short stature. Other symptoms include osteoporosis, curvature of the spine (scoliosis), rickets, excessive mobility of joints (hypermobility), joint swelling and arthritis, and weak or absent deep tendon reflexes (areflexia). Those affected by this disorder experience gastro-oesophageal reflux, a condition in which the stomach contents flow back into the oesophagus, and kidney problems, including a loss of bicarbonate, sodium, potassium, amino and organic acids, calcium, phosphate and L-carnitine in the urine (Fanconi-type renal tubular dysfunction). Facial characteristics include deep-set eyes, a long face, a prominent forehead and dental problems. Affected individuals also have learning disabilities, behavioural problems, feeding difficulties, seizures, underdeveloped testes and, in some cases, constipation.

Lowe syndrome can be diagnosed on the basis of skin tests, enzyme deficiency and DNA analysis, and study of tissue samples to identify abnormalities of the kidney, testes and/or brain. A specialised eye examination may determine whether a female is a carrier of the disorder. Prenatal diagnosis is available. Treatment of this disorder is dependent upon symptoms. Kidney problems relating to a lack of phosphorus can be managed by oral replacement therapy, and sodium bicarbonate can reduce the accumulation of acid in the blood and urine. Consultation with a paediatric ophthalmologist and a glaucoma specialist is recommended for individuals with cataracts and glaucoma. Surgery is necessary for the removal of cataracts, and should be undertaken at an early age in order to maintain visual stimulation and development. Replacement lenses are not recommended, due to the high incidence of glaucoma. Visual aids may also be helpful. Feeding tubes or a gastrostomy may be necessary in order to overcome feeding difficulties. Gastro-oesophageal reflux usually responds to measures such as thickened feedings and elevation of the head of the child's bed. Some patients may need medication to control stomach acid production and to aid emptying of the stomach, while others may need surgery. Human growth hormone therapy has been successful in improving growth velocity. Surgery or bracing may be required to correct severe scoliosis and joint hypermobility. Anti-convulsant therapy may be necessary to control seizures. Vitamin D supplements may be used to prevent rickets. Special programmes should be started in early infancy to aid the child's development. Physiotherapy, occupational therapy, visual impairment services, special education and speech and language therapy are all included in these programmes, which are planned around the needs of the individual.

Reviewed by the Lowe Syndrome Trust, UK

Russell–Silver syndrome

Other names for this condition

- RSS
- Russell–Silver dwarfism
- Russell–Silver syndrome, X-linked (Partington syndrome)
- Russell syndrome
- Silver syndrome
- Silver–Russell dwarfism
- Silver–Russell syndrome
- Silver's asymmetry–dwarfism

Russell–Silver syndrome is a rare disorder that is characterised by a short length measurement and a low weight at birth, usually accompanied by a long narrow head. This disorder is occasionally caused by a genetic mutation involving a gene located on the long arm of chromosome 7. Usually one pair of a set of chromosomes is inherited from the mother, and another is inherited from the father. In a small number (about 10%) of patients with Russell–Silver syndrome, both number 7 chromosomes are inherited from the mother, and this is described as 'disomy from chromosome 7.' Interestingly, these patients tend to be at the mild end of the Russell–Silver syndrome spectrum, and do not have limb asymmetry. There are also other abnormalities which have been described on chromosome 11.

Symptoms of this disorder may vary widely, and usually include a triangular-shaped face (this shape lessens with age), growth problems, poor appetite in the early years, and curvature of the fifth finger (clinodactyly). Other symptoms include low blood sugar levels (hypoglycaemia) in infancy and early childhood, an overgrowth of limbs on one side of the body (asymmetry), and late closure of the fontanelle. In addition, there may be facial abnormalities such as a broad, prominent forehead, a small chin, a thin upper lip, downturned corners of the mouth, small crowded teeth and abnormal ears. Those affected may also have a high-pitched voice, fused or webbed toes, an abnormal location of the urethral opening (hypospadius), unde-scended testicles, delayed bone age, weak muscle tone and developmental delay.

Diagnosis of Russell–Silver syndrome is made on the basis of detection of the symptoms. No tests to aid diagnosis are available at present. Treatment of the disorder is largely dependent on symptoms, and may include a change in diet, use of a feeding pump and/or a gastrostomy, which helps to increase the calorie intake. Ear tubes are sometimes used to improve fluid drainage from the ears. Shoe lifts and limb-lengthening surgery may be used to help to correct asymmetry. Paediatric dentists can help to manage dental problems, and surgery is not usually needed for this. Speech therapy and physiotherapy are also of benefit. Genetic counselling is recommended for individuals affected by this disorder.

Reviewed by Dr R Stanhope

Velocardiofacial syndrome

Other names for this condition
- 22q11 deletion syndrome
- Shprintzen syndrome
- VCFS
- DiGeorge syndrome

Velocardiofacial syndrome consists of three symptoms, namely congenital heart abnormalities, cleft palate (a gap in the roof of the mouth) and a characteristic facial appearance. In almost all affected individuals, genetic studies show that a piece of chromosome 22 is missing by fluorescence *in-situ* hybridisation (FISH) analysis. This is known as the 22q11 deletion, which occurs 1 in 4000 members of the population.

In most cases, velocardiofacial syndrome occurs sporadically for no known reason. However, this condition is inherited in an autosomal dominant manner in around 10–15% of cases.

Velocardiofacial syndrome may present before birth on routine antenatal ultrasound scanning, or at birth or shortly afterwards, with symptoms caused by a structural abnormality of the heart. Feeding difficulties due to a cleft palate, or weakness and disproportion of the palate resulting in failure to close the space between the back of the mouth and the nose (a condition known as velopharyngeal disproportion or VPI), may also present early. If the palate is not obviously cleft, the condition may not be recognised until childhood. Slow development, especially of speech, is apparent after 1 year of age, and learning disorders may become noticeable in nursery school, at normal school age or in adulthood.

The symptoms of velocardiofacial syndrome vary widely. Nasal regurgitation, difficulty in swallowing and chewing, and later the nasal escape of air during speech are characteristic of a cleft palate or VPI. Breathlessness and cyanosis (bluish-purple discoloration of the skin) may be due to abnormalities of the heart, which mainly affect the wall separating the right and left chambers of the heart, the large arteries coming out of the heart, and the circulation to the lungs. Other symptoms include learning difficulties, immune system problems and loss of muscle tone. The appearance of affected individuals is often characterised by a broad nasal bridge, narrow nostrils, narrow eyelids, blue shadows underneath the eyes, prominent ears (often of different size) with thickened outer rims, small stature, tapered hands and a small-sized head (microcephaly). Many affected children also have frequent ear infections and recurrent chest infections. Unrecognised hypocalcaemia can be associated with seizures. The kidneys may be affected by infection, or on ultrasound examination they may show cysts or a baggy collecting system, or a single kidney may be found.

Behaviour can be affected by symptoms of attention deficit, autistic features, rapid cycles of mood, panicky feelings, and in young adults an increased likelihood of schizophrenia.

There are approximately 180 abnormalities caused by the deletion, although the severity and number of symptoms vary widely from one individual to another.

Treatment for velocardiofacial syndrome is dependent on the severity of various symptoms. Surgical repair of the more severe heart defects, and cleft palate, is usually undertaken in infancy. In childhood, surgery may be required to correct the heart, to help to improve speech if VPI is present, and to improve hearing by inserting air-ventilating tubes (grommets) in the ears. In addition to a heart examination, it is usual to check the kidneys, the blood calcium levels and the immune system so that appropriate advice on vaccinations can be given. It is also very likely that a range of specialists will be called in to talk to the parents.

Research into velocardiofacial syndrome is ongoing.

Reviewed by Dr A Habel

X-linked hypophosphataemic rickets

> **Other names for this condition**
> - XLHR

Rickets is a bone-softening condition of childhood caused by inadequate mineralisation of the growth plate due to a deficiency of calcium and phosphorus. This leads to deformity and impaired growth of long bones. The commonest cause of rickets world-wide is vitamin D deficiency, which in turn leads to impaired absorption of calcium from the diet. In some African and South Asian countries, dietary deficiency of calcium is the most important cause of rickets. The adult form of rickets is known as osteomalacia.

A number of inherited conditions that cause low blood levels of phosphorus (hypophosphataemia) as a result of increased loss of this mineral in the urine can also cause rickets and osteomalacia. The commonest form of familial hypo-phosphataemic rickets is X-linked hypophosphataemic rickets (XLHR). An affected father will pass the disease on to all of his daughters, whereas an affected mother has a 50% chance of passing the disease on to her offspring of either sex. Most patients with XLHR have been shown to have mutations in the *PHEX* gene (a phosphateregulating gene with homologies to endopeptidases on the X chromosome). This gene has been localised to the Xp22.1 position on the short arm of the X chromosome. The product of the *PHEX* gene interacts with other factors, such as fibroblastic growth factor 23 (FGF23), to prevent loss of phosphorus in the urine, and also helps to maintain normal blood levels of the active form of vitamin D (1,25-dihydroxyvitamin D_3). Other conditions that lead to hypophosphataemic rickets include autosomal-domin-ant hypophosphataemic rickets, hereditary hypophosphataemic rickets with hyper-calciuria, and tumour-induced rickets.

Children with XLHR tend to develop bowed legs at the time of weight bearing. They often walk with a waddling and intoeing gait. Short stature with disproportionate shortening of the lower limbs is an important clinical feature in an untreated child. Patients with this condition often develop dental abscesses in the absence of dental caries. Premature closure of the cranial sutures (gaps between the bones of the skull) may lead to distortion of the skull shape and occasionally symptoms and signs of raised pressure within the skull (raised intracranial pressure). Some adults with XLHR show calcification of spinal ligaments and narrowing of the spinal canal.

The diagnosis can usually be made on the basis of a thorough clinical assessment, skeletal radiographs (X-ray films) and appropriate blood and urine analysis. The treatment of XLHR should be undertaken by a specialist with expertise in the assessment and treatment of bone disorders. At present it involves ingestion of oral phosphate supplements 4 to 6 times a day and medication in the form of calcitriol or alfacalcidol, taken once or twice a day. Careful monitoring of treatment is necessary in order to avoid secondary complications, such as hyperparathyroidism, and calcium deposits in the kidney (nephrocalcinosis). Patients also require regular dental care because of the risk of developing spontaneous dental abscesses. In some adolescents surgery to correct limb deformities may be necessary.

Reviewed by Dr Z Mughal

Chapter 9

Blood and immune system disorders

Blood disorders

The blood disorders include a number of different types of disorder. The majority of the disorders in the group are bleeding disorders, such as the factor deficiencies. Blood coagulation factors enable the blood to clot by producing fibrin, a protein that is produced in order to stop bleeding. If there is a deficiency of one of the factors, bleeding becomes a problem following injury or surgery, and can also cause other complications. Other blood disorders in this group include red blood cell abnormalities, defects of the blood vessels, and disorders due to impaired production of haemoglobin or destruction of red blood cells.

Immune system disorders

The immune system defends the body against harmful substances (antigens) such as bacteria, viruses and foreign bodies by producing antibodies in response to these antigens. Immune system disorders occur when the immune response is impaired and the body is left vulnerable to infections. Immunodeficiency disorders occur when all or part of the immune system fails. Autoimmune disorders occur when the immune system acts to destroy the body's own cells and tissues.

Acrodermatitis enteropathica

Other names for this condition

- AE
- Brandt syndrome
- Danbolt–Cross syndrome
- Zinc deficiency, congenital

There are two forms of this condition, an acquired form and a form that is apparent at birth (a congenital form). The acquired form is due to insufficient zinc in the diet. In the congenital form, there appears to be a deficiency or an absence of a zinc transporter in the intestines, which can lead to zinc malabsorption and a deficiency of zinc. There is also a deficiency of the enzyme alkaline phosphatase, which is a consequence of zinc deficiency.

This disorder is genetically inherited from the parents in an autosomal recessive manner.

Symptoms of this condition appear gradually during the first few weeks of life if a baby is breastfed. This is because breast milk contains low levels of zinc. If a baby is bottle fed, symptoms tend to appear around the time of weaning. The main symptom is usually inflammation of the skin, with pimples that often blister and then dry up to form scaly red patches. The areas of skin that tend to be affected are around the mouth, bottom and eyes and on the elbows, knees, hands and feet. Other symptoms may include chronic diarrhoea, loose bulky stools due to the presence of fatty substances in the stools (steatorrhoea), inflammation around the nails, hair loss on the scalp, eyelids and eyebrows, and inflammation of the membrane around the eyes (conjunctivitis).

In the acute phase of this disorder, irritability and emotional disturbances may occur due to wasting (atrophy) of the outer membrane of the brain. Zinc levels in the blood may be abnormally low, due to lack of a zinc-binding factor that is normally produced by the pancreas. Infants who are breastfed by a mother who has acrodermatitis enteropathica may have low levels of zinc in their blood with other symptoms of this disorder, due to a deficiency of the zinc-binding factor in the mother's milk.

This disorder is treated with zinc supplements (zinc sulphate), which should be continued for life. Each individual may require slightly different levels of supplements, and these should be given as soon as the diagnosis has been confirmed. Foods with a high zinc content may be helpful. These include oysters, beef, liver, pumpkin seeds, pecans and brazil nuts. Diodoquin (iodoquinol) is a drug that may be used to treat this disorder. It usually clears up the symptoms of the disorder within a week. Remission of the condition commonly occurs during puberty, but it may recur in some women during pregnancy. Genetic counselling is recommended for those affected by this disorder.

Reviewed by Dr MJ Henderson

Alpha-1-antitrypsin deficiency

Other names for this condition

- A1AD
- A1AT deficiency
- Alpha-1-ATD
- Antitrypsin deficiency
- Neonatal cholestasis
- Familial chronic obstructive lung disease
- Familial emphysema
- Hereditary emphysema
- Homozygous alpha-1-antitrypsin deficiency
- PI
- Pi phenotype ZZ or Z- and Z-
- Protease inhibitor deficiency
- Serum protease inhibitor deficiency

Alpha-1-antitrypsin deficiency is a disorder characterised by low levels or an absence of a protein known as alpha-1-antitrypsin, which is produced by the liver and then released into the bloodstream. Alpha-1-antitrypsin protects the lungs from damage by enzymes known as proteases. A deficiency can result in breathing difficulties and causes the air sacs in the lungs to become enlarged and damaged. The disorder may lead to emphysema and liver disease (cirrhosis).

This disorder is genetically inherited from the parents in an autosomal recessive manner.

Symptoms of the disorder may include jaundice (yellowing of the skin) in the neonatal period, high blood pressure in the portal vein (portal hypertension), enlargement of the liver and/or spleen, persistent yellow-coloured urine, pale stools, accumulation of fluid in the body (ascites) and poor weight gain. Other symptoms include unintentional weight loss, excessive thirst, breathing difficulties, headache, mood swings, fatigue, insomnia, impaired concentration, memory loss, agitation and lethargy. Affected individuals may have swollen legs, feet and ankles, chest abnormalities, a swollen abdomen, and a rash or open sores on the hands and feet. They may also be pale, have a rapid heartbeat, feel dizzy or faint when standing, and have impaired judgement. Other symptoms include vomiting (the vomit may contain blood), abnormal bowel movements and problems with vision. In later life, this disorder can cause emphysema, which is a chronic progressive illness that may include a chronic cough, production of phlegm and some wheezing. In other cases, individuals at any stage between infancy and adulthood may present with inflammation of the liver (hepatitis).

This disorder can be diagnosed by blood tests that measure the level of alpha-1-antitrypsin and the phenotype in the blood. A good diet, exercise and the avoidance of smoking and alcohol will increase the likelihood of long-term health. Prolastin treatment is effective for lung disease, and antibiotics may be used to treat infections. A lung transplant may be necessary in some cases. The liver and lung symptoms can be treated with medication. Symptomatic treatment for liver problems is required, and a transplant may be necessary. Enzyme replacement therapy for this disorder is available.

Reviewed by Professor DA Kelly

Ataxia telangiectasia

> **Other names for this condition**
> - AT
> - Cerebello-oculocutaneous telangiectasia
> - Immunodeficiency with ataxia telangiectasia
> - Louis–Bar syndrome

This is a slow progressive disorder that affects the brain, causing an inability to coordinate muscle movements (ataxia). Ataxia telangiectasia is caused by a deficiency of the ataxia–telangiectasia-mutated (ATM) protein that plays a role in preventing the division of cells following damage to the DNA. If there is a deficiency of the protein the cells continue to divide and the DNA is not repaired. The ATM protein deficiency is caused by a defect in the *ATM* gene that is located on the long arm of chromosome 11.

This disorder is genetically inherited from the parents in an autosomal recessive manner.

The symptoms of this condition usually present during infancy or childhood. They commonly include tremors due to involuntary muscle contractions, and a progressive loss of the ability to coordinate muscle movements (ataxia), leading to a loss of ability to walk by late childhood or adolescence. The affected individual may exhibit slow writhing or jerky movements. At the age of around 3 to 6 years there is characteristically development of red lesions on the skin and mucous membranes of the eye, due to the permanent widening of groups of blood vessels (telangiectasia). There may also be difficulty in coordinating certain eye movements, as well as rapid involuntary movements of the eye. Affected individuals have an impaired immune system, which makes them more susceptible to infections. The latter can be serious and may be life threatening. Other symptoms may include growth delay, premature ageing, incomplete sexual development, nosebleeds, absence of the tonsils, and poor muscle coordination in the head and neck, causing speech problems, swallowing difficulties and choking. In addition, individuals who have this disorder or who are carriers seem to be at increased risk of developing cancers. The exposure to X-rays may increase the incidence of possible tumours. In some cases, individuals affected by this disorder develop a mild form of diabetes mellitus.

Ataxia telangiectasia can be diagnosed on the basis of a physical examination, a medical family history and a range of tests, including an MRI scan, blood tests and a specialised test to demonstrate chromosome abnormalities (karyotyping). Treatment for individuals with this disorder aims to relieve any symptoms and provide support in the care of the individual. Physical and occupational therapy may help to maintain flexibility. As affected individuals have a weakened immune system, antibiotics should be given promptly for infections, and gammaglobulin injections may also be beneficial. Reducing exposure to sunlight will help to prevent the spread of skin lesions. Vitamin E may be of some benefit, and diazepam may aid speech problems and muscle contractions. Affected individuals rarely survive beyond their mid-twenties, due to their weakened immune system. Genetic counselling is recommended for those affected by this disorder.

Reviewed by Dr MA McShane

Blue rubber bleb naevus syndrome

Other names for this condition
- Bean syndrome
- BRBNS

Blue rubber bleb naevus syndrome is a rare disorder of the venous blood vessels. It is characterised by multiple soft raised nodules on the skin or just beneath it. The nodules contain blood vessels, which can give them a blue colour, and are soft to the touch. This condition was first reported by Dr William Bean, who said that these small lumps had the look and feel of a 'rubber nipple.' The nodules can vary in colour, size, shape and number, and may be tender. They may not only be present in the skin but also in the mouth, the conjunctiva (the white of the eye) and on internal organs, including the intestines, liver, lungs and brain. If they are present in the intestines, gastrointestinal bleeding is common, and this can cause a low blood count (anaemia).

In some cases, blue rubber bleb naevus syndrome can result from genetic changes that appear to occur for no reason. However, in other cases this disorder is inherited within a family in an autosomal dominant manner.

The lesions can appear at birth or in early childhood, and may increase in size and frequency with age. Oral cavity haemangiomas occur in 60% of cases. The skin nodules are typically located on the upper arms or trunk of the body, and may be surrounded by areas of excessive sweating (hyperhidrosis). They are also found internally in many different areas, including the liver, kidney, spleen, gallbladder, lungs and muscles. Complications of this disorder include internal haemorrhaging. If nodules are located in the brain, they may cause haemorrhaging and increased pressure on the brain. Rarely, blue rubber bleb naevi have been reported in a few patients who have had growths in other tissues, such as the bone, cartilage, lymphatic system and the brain, that have not resulted from abnormal blood vessels.

All treatment of this disorder aims to relieve symptoms and provide support in the care of the individual. Anaemic patients may require iron supplements and blood transfusions. In cases where there is repeated bleeding from the intestines, laser surgery may be successful, although surgical removal of the nodules may sometimes be indicated.

Reviewed by Dr A Fryer

Factor X deficiency

> **Other names for this condition**
> - FX deficiency
> - Stuart–Prower deficiency

The factor deficiencies are a group of blood coagulation (clotting) disorders. The blood clotting process uses up to 20 different plasma proteins, which are also known as blood coagulation factors. These factors are involved in forming a protein known as fibrin, which is produced in order to stop bleeding. Factor X deficiency is a rare disorder characterised by abnormal blood coagulation that is caused by a deficiency of the plasma protein factor X.

This disorder can be caused by amyloidosis, in which protein fibres are deposited in the organs and muscles (*see* p. 111 for a summary). Factor X deficiency can also be genetically inherited from the parents in an autosomal recessive manner.

Symptoms of this disorder include nosebleeds, excessive bruising, bleeding of the mucous membranes, excessive menstrual bleeding, bleeding from the umbilical cord stump, and bleeding in the mother after the delivery of a baby. There may be bleeding into the brain, the joints (haemarthrosis) and the muscles and/or body tissues (haematomas). If such bleeding is frequent or left untreated, it can cause permanent damage. There may be prolonged bleeding if an injury occurs, and during and after surgery. Newborn males who are circumcised may also experience prolonged bleeding. There may be an accumulation of blood in the gut, and blood may also be found in the urine (haematuria). Affected individuals may experience miscarriage during the first trimester. As with most of the factor deficiencies, the severity of the bleeding depends on the level of factor X – the lower the level, the more serious the bleeding problems will be.

Factor X deficiency can be diagnosed in the newborn period if the baby has a bleeding episode. In some cases the disorder is diagnosed later in life when the patient shows signs of abnormal bleeding. Blood samples are taken to measure the amount of time it takes for the blood to clot. The blood test can demonstrate the factor X deficiency. Treatment of this disorder includes the administration of infusions of frozen blood plasma or concentrates that contain factor X during acute episodes or in preparation for surgery. Bleeding in the brain can be life threatening, and medical treatment should be sought immediately if this is suspected. Major muscle bleeds can cause permanent muscle damage, so it is important to seek medical advice in this situation. Treatment for individuals with factor X deficiency related to amyloidosis involves surgical removal of the spleen. Vitamin K supplements may be recommended, and a reduction in the intake of alcohol is also advised, to reduce the risk of liver disease. The prognosis for individuals with this disorder is generally good.

Reviewed by Dr D Keeling

Gilbert syndrome

Other names for this condition

- Constitutional liver dysfunction
- Familial jaundice
- Gilbert's disease
- Gilbert–Lereboullet syndrome
- Hyperbilirubinaemia I
- Hyperbilirubinemia, Arias type
- Icterus intermittens juvenalis
- Meulengracht's disease
- Unconjugated benign bilirubinaemia

Gilbert syndrome is a disorder that results in impairment of the removal of bile pigment (bilirubin) from the liver. It is characterised by jaundice that is most evident on the face, the palms of the hands and the soles of the feet. This is a result of an abnormal increase in bilirubin levels in the blood. This disorder is thought to be caused by decreased activity of an enzyme system known as bilirubin-uridine diphosphate glucuronyl transferase (bilirubin-UGT). The gene responsible for this disorder is located on the long arm of chromosome 2.

The disorder is inherited in an autosomal dominant fashion.

Gilbert syndrome is a mild condition that appears to affect males more than females. Symptoms appear shortly after birth, but may not be recognised. Mild jaundice, which is more common in males, appears at the age of around 10 years, and may increase in response to stress, strain or exposure to low temperatures. The whites of the eyes may also appear yellow. Other symptoms may include fatigue, nausea, loss of appetite, weakness, abdominal pain and (rarely) diarrhoea and enlargement of the liver and spleen. Some of these symptoms may be provoked by dehydration, missing meals, repeated vomiting, fever, menstruation and vigorous exercise. Yellow spots and marks similar to moles may be noticeable on the eyelids, and the skin pigment may change as a result of exposure to light and heat.

Diagnosis can be made on the basis of a blood test that measures the activity of the defective enzyme. However, this test is not widely available. A doctor commonly gives patients with jaundice a simple blood test to make sure that the cause is not serious. If repeated blood tests show increased levels of bilirubin, it is likely that the patient has Gilbert syndrome. Other tests to confirm the diagnosis may include a urine test, physical examination and a detailed patient history.

Treatment of this disorder may include phenobarbital, which controls jaundice and reduces the levels of bilirubin. However, this drug is only used if the doctor feels that the bilirubin levels are becoming too high. Individuals affected by this disorder must be careful to control their diet, as missing meals can lead to elevated levels of bilirubin. This disorder causes no harm, and treatment is usually unnecessary. Patients who are diagnosed with this disorder should be reassured that they will be able to lead normal lives and that the prognosis is excellent.

Reviewed by Professor DA Kelly

Glucose-6-phosphate dehydrogenase deficiency

Other names for this condition

- Favism
- G6PD deficiency

In this disorder there is a deficiency of the enzyme glucose-6-phosphate dehydrogenase. This enzyme is required to form glutathione, an antioxidant that is needed to protect the red blood cells which transport oxygen around the body using haemoglobin. If there are insufficient levels of the antioxidant glutathione, premature destruction of red blood cells will occur. This process of destruction is stimulated when individuals are exposed to certain medications, chemicals, viruses, bacterial infections, or the pollen of or food products containing fava beans (broad beans). One benefit of having this disorder is that it confers a resistance to developing malaria.

Glucose-6-phosphate dehydrogenase deficiency is inherited from the parents in an X-linked fashion. This disorder occurs more frequently in individuals from South-East Asia, Africa, the Middle East and areas of the Mediterranean. For further information about the inheritance of this disorder, a genetic counselling service should be consulted.

Symptoms vary widely from one individual to another. This is because there are thought to be over 300 different variants. The condition may initially present at birth with yellowing of the skin (jaundice) that persists beyond normal. In a small number of individuals the jaundice can be severe, and may cause brain damage and in some cases can even be fatal. Other symptoms commonly appear following exposure to the above-mentioned factors. These may include fatigue, pallor, shortness of breath, rapid heartbeat (tachycardia), yellowing of the skin (jaundice), fever, dark urine, an enlarged spleen (splenomegaly), pains in the back and abdomen and dizziness.

Individuals with this disorder should avoid being treated with certain drugs, eating fava beans or being exposed to areas where fava beans are grown (because of the pollen) in order to prevent episodes of haemolytic anaemia. There are many different variants of the disorder, so the effects of different medications vary from one individual to another, and some individuals are less sensitive to fava beans (broad beans). If symptoms occur, the affected individual should see a doctor, as these episodes can be life threatening and treatment is required. If the episode occurs in response to a medication, this must be stopped under the supervision of a doctor, and if it is due to an infection, this must be treated. Oxygen, fluids and sometimes blood transfusions are also needed. Neonatal jaundice is treated by using special lights to help to break down the bilirubin that causes yellowing of the skin.

Reviewed by Dr C Lambert

Turner syndrome

Other names for this condition

- 45,X syndrome
- Bonnevie–Ulrich syndrome
- Gonadal dysgenesis
- Gonadal dysgenesis
- Monosomy X
- Morgagni–Turner–Albright syndrome
- Ovarian dwarfism, Turner type
- Ovary aplasia, Turner type
- Pterygolymphangiectasia
- Schereshevkii–Turner syndrome
- TS
- Turner–Varny syndrome
- XO syndrome

Turner syndrome is a rare disorder that occurs only in females. It is characterised by the complete or partial absence of one of the X chromosomes. The X chromosomes carry genes for ovary development and oestrogen production, so a deficiency causes many women to become infertile, and have faulty development of the ovaries and various other problems. Symptoms vary with regard to how many cells are affected by the changes to the chromosome.

The exact cause of Turner syndrome is unknown. However, it is believed that it may be caused by an error during the division of the parents' sex cells. The X and Y chromosomes (known as sex chromosomes) are responsible for determining the sex of the child. When eggs or sperm are formed, a sex chromosome may go missing or become partially absent. When this happens, a male embryo will only receive the Y chromosome and will not survive. However, if the female embryo receives one X chromosome she may survive and develop Turner syndrome. In some cases the disorder may be caused by defects in the X chromosome, or the chromosome may disappear during the development of the embryo, affecting certain cells that are needed for development.

Symptoms of this disorder include abnormal body proportions, growth delay, and lack of a 'growth spurt' during puberty. The average adult height for women with Turner syndrome is between 4ft 5in and 4ft 8in (approx. 1.37m and 1.46m respectively). Women with this disorder also have undeveloped breasts, a delayed or absent menstrual cycle, and an absence of pubic or underarm hair. Some women may have characteristic facial features, including a small jaw (micrognathia) that is abnormally low, droopy eyelids (ptosis), prominent low-set ears, a high narrow palate and a low hairline at the front and back. Affected individuals may have heart defects, including contraction of the large artery in the heart (aortic constriction). Other symptoms include a broad chest, swelling of the hands and feet (lymphoedema), elbow malformations, a large number of moles, loose skin folds on the neck and shoulders, unusually shaped kidneys and an extra set of urethras. Those affected may also suffer from disorientation and hearing difficulties.

This disorder can be diagnosed on the basis of a specialised blood test that can detect the absence or partial absence of the X chromosome. Treatment of this disorder involves oestrogen therapy from a young age and the administration of a recombinant human growth hormone from the age of 7 years through to puberty, when oestrogen replacement therapy may be started. *In-vitro* fertilisation (IVF) is sometimes possible. The growth hormones Humatrope[R] and Nutropin have been approved by the US Food and Drug Administration for use in this condition.

Research into treatment for this disorder is ongoing.

Reviewed by Dr K Lachlan

Von Willebrand disease

Other names for this condition

- Angiohaemophilia
- Constitutional thrombopathy
- Minot–Von Willebrand disease
- Pseudohaemophilia
- Vascular haemophilia
- Von Willebrand factor deficiency
- VWD
- Willebrand–Juergans disease

Von Willebrand disease (VWD) is a genetic disorder that affects the ability of the blood to clot properly. It is mainly characterised by prolonged bleeding and vulnerability to bruising. All types of Von Willebrand disease are caused by problems with the Von Willebrand factor (VWF) protein. The main function of VWF is to support the blood's platelets, which therefore cannot function properly in VWD. The VWF protein also helps to protect factor VIII, a blood-clotting factor. The gene for VWF is located on the short arm of chromosome 12.

There are various types of Von Willebrand disease.

- Type 1 is the mildest form of this disorder. The level of VWF is reduced, but symptoms may be very mild. Aspirin and other non-steroidal anti-inflammatory drugs may worsen this condition.
- Type 2A – the particles that make up the VWF are smaller than usual and can break down too easily.
- Type 2B – the VWF sticks too firmly to platelet cells which help to repair torn blood vessels. This leads to platelets becoming clustered, which results in a low platelet number.
- Type 3 – patients experience severe bleeding problems.
- Pseudo or platelet type – this is similar to type 2B, but the platelets rather than the VWF are defective.

This disorder is inherited in an autosomal dominant manner.

Symptoms of this disorder usually appear in infancy or early childhood, and include an increased risk of excessive bleeding following surgery, injury, menstruation and/or childbirth. In the rare type 3 disease, internal bleeding into the joints may occur. Those who are severely affected may experience heavy bleeding into the mucous membrane and into the passage from the oesophagus through to the large intestine. This is fairly common, but may be life threatening. Other symptoms include common nosebleeds, skin rash and bleeding gums.

Von Willebrand disease can be diagnosed on the basis of clinical tests to determine VWF levels, and monitoring of the bleeding time. These tests may need to be repeated due to changes in the levels of substances in the blood. Treatment of the type 1 disorder includes desmopressin, a synthetic drug that is a copy of a hormone. Cyklokapron® and Amicar® are other useful drugs that help to hold a clot in place once it has formed. Other treatments include a factor VIII concentrate that contains Von Willebrand factor. This is used for the type 3 disorder, serious bleeding or major surgery, and occasionally for some cases of the type 2 disorder. In addition, cryoprecipitate is a blood component that can be used to control excess bleeding. Dosages must be monitored to avoid any other complications, activities that carry a high risk of injury should be avoided, and it is recommended that those affected should have a precautionary immunisation against hepatitis B.

Research into this condition is ongoing.

Reviewed by Dr D Keeling

Wiskott–Aldrich syndrome

Other names for this condition

- Aldrich syndrome
- IMD2
- Immunodeficiency 2
- Immunodeficiency with thrombocytopenia and eczema
- WAS

This is a disorder that affects the immune system and causes individuals to become susceptible to infections. This is due to defects in T-lymphocytes and B-lymphocytes. The T-cells are responsible for fighting yeast, fungi, viruses and bacteria, whereas the B-cells fight infection caused by bacteria. The B-cells work by producing antibodies that either directly kill microorganisms or cover them so that they are more easily destroyed by other white blood cells. As there is a deficiency of both B- and T-cells, this condition is classed as a combined immunodeficiency (CID). Because the defects leave some cell functions intact, affected individuals are susceptible to infection by certain types of microorganisms, but may be protected against other microorganisms.

This disorder is inherited in an X-linked manner.

Symptoms usually present soon after birth or during the first year of life with a combination of recurrent infection, low levels of platelets in the blood, eczema and autoimmune symptoms. Individuals with Wiskott–Aldrich syndrome are particularly prone to recurrent infections of the middle ear (otitis media), inflammation of the lungs (pneumonia) and sometimes inflammation of the membranes that protect the brain and spinal cord (meningitis). Another symptom is a reduced number of platelets in the blood (thrombocytopenia). Platelets are cells in the blood that help to stop bleeding. The lack of platelets is due to the fact that they have an abnormal shape (they are also very small) and are removed from the blood by the spleen. Low numbers of platelets can cause small purple spots on the skin from small bleeds below the skin's surface (petechiae), as well as blood in the stools, bleeding gums, prolonged nosebleeds and an enlarged spleen (splenomegaly).

Further complications may include the risk of bleeding into the brain after a bump on the head. Frequently there are also scaly and itchy skin rashes (eczema). In infants, this may appear as thick yellow patchy scabs on the head (cradle cap) and/or inflammation and irritation of the skin in the nappy area (nappy rash). In older children, eczema tends to occur in creases around the knees, elbows, wrists and neck. Autoimmune symptoms occur when the immune system reacts against part of an individual's own body. Symptoms may include high fever without an infection with possible rashes, painful swelling of the joints, and swelling of areas of the legs that are not associated with the joints. In addition, there may be a further decrease in the number of platelets (which can be life threatening if bleeding occurs), anaemia may occur due to blood loss from the digestive system or due to the destruction of red blood cells, and there may be inflammation of the arteries in different parts of the body. Some affected individuals are also prone to developing certain types of cancers, such as lymphoma and leukaemia.

Patients with Wiskott–Aldrich syndrome show wide variation in the level of symptoms, ranging from the severally affected to those with moderate symptoms. Treatments are based on the severity of the symptoms and the individual options for treatment. This disorder can be treated with a bone-marrow transplant using a donor who is tissue (HLA) compatible, often a sibling but occasionally a matched unrelated donor. HLA matching helps to prevent the recipient tissue from being recognised as foreign by the donor cells. A bone-marrow transplant will cure this disorder. An alternative procedure is an umbilical cord stem-cell transfusion, which can also cure the syndrome. In individuals for whom these procedures are unsuitable, the removal of the spleen will in most cases stop the destruction of platelets and help to maintain normal levels of platelets in the blood. This means that the individual will be able to participate in some physical activities that would otherwise need to be avoided if platelet counts are very low. Often regular antibiotic medications are given, as well as antibodies (gammaglobins) to help to prevent infections. In some cases, platelet transfusions are given to raise platelet levels. Gene therapy for this disorder is under development, and if successful would also cure this condition.

When infections occur, prompt treatment is required with the necessary antibiotics. Individuals with this disorder should not be given live virus vaccines, as these may lead to the disease that the patient has been vaccinated against, as their immune systems will be susceptible to certain microorganisms. However, other household members should be vaccinated so that they do not bring home infections. The regular use of moisturising cream and avoidance of excessive bathing (which dries out the skin) can help eczema. Steroid creams may be used sparingly on areas of chronic inflammation. It should be noted that certain foods can make eczema worse. Autoimmune symptoms may require steroid treatment or other immunosuppressive drugs, but these should only be used if the symptoms are severe, as they can further depress immune function. Diseases such as chickenpox can be life threatening to individuals who are taking steroids.

Reviewed by Dr KC Gilmour

Chapter 10

Associated disorders

The 'associated disorders' represent a group that has been set up to incorporate the large number of disorders on which Climb holds information for various reasons.

The group includes disorders that are:

- of an unknown cause
- suspected to be metabolic
- closely related to a metabolic disorder
- rare and for which there is little information and support available, and Climb is the only point of contact available.

Bloom syndrome

Other names for this condition

- BS

Bloom syndrome is a rare genetic disorder caused by a defect in the gene that codes for the BLM protein (DNA helicase RecQ protein-like-3). The role of the protein is not known. This disorder is more prevalent in the Eastern European Ashkenazi Jewish population.

Bloom syndrome is genetically inherited from the parents in an autosomal recessive manner.

The main symptoms of this disorder include an abnormally short stature, sensitivity to light (photosensitivity), and a number of small dilated blood vessels on the face, especially on the cheeks and nose (facial telangiectasia). Babies may appear small at birth. Children with the disorder may have a small narrow head and face with flat cheekbones and, in some cases, prominent ears and nose. The skin may have dark patches known as café-au-lait spots, which can be found anywhere on the body. Affected individuals are prone to infections and respiratory difficulties due to a deficiency of the immune system, and have a higher susceptibility to cancer of any organ. Cancers may develop very early in life, often in childhood, with a mean age at diagnosis of about 25 years. Many individuals develop a malignant tumour, especially leukaemia, and some may also develop diabetes. Other symptoms can include diarrhoea, vomiting, increased sweating, dental abnormalities, inflammation of the lips (cheilitis), a high-pitched voice, cysts on the spine, and abnormalities of the eyes, ears, feet and hands, including extra digits. Males are infertile and unable to produce sperm, and females have a lowered fertility because they may cease menstruation at an abnormally young age. Some individuals may have learning difficulties and developmental delay.

This disorder can be diagnosed on the basis of a laboratory test known as a chromosome study to show the exchanges and abnormalities in the chromosomes of individuals suspected of having the disorder. Treatment for individuals with this disease aims to relieve any symptoms and provide support in the care of the individual. Those who are affected should check for signs of cancer on a regular basis. Antibiotics may help to clear up any infections. Affected individuals should avoid direct contact with sunlight, and sunscreen should be of benefit. A dermatologist should be consulted on a regular basis.

Reviewed by Professor ID Hickson

Cockayne syndrome

Other names for this condition

- CS
- Deafness–dwarfism–retinal atrophy
- Dwarfism with renal atrophy and deafness
- Neill–Dingwall syndrome
- Progeroid nanism

This disorder is a metabolic disease that is characterised by restricted growth, sensitivity to light and premature ageing. Cockayne syndrome is thought to develop as a result of the DNA's inability to repair damage caused by exposure to ultraviolet light, which is a component of sunlight.

There are three types of Cockayne syndrome:

- type 1 – the classical form in which symptoms are progressive and appear around the age of 1 year
- type 2 – the congenital form in which symptoms are present at birth
- type 3 – the late-onset form in which symptoms begin later in life.

This disorder is genetically inherited from the parents in an autosomal recessive manner.

In all three types of this disorder the symptoms are similar, with only the age of onset varying. The main effects of this syndrome are the stunting of growth, with affected individuals having disproportionately longer arms and legs, and large hands and feet. Children may be extremely sensitive to light (photosensitive) and develop sunburn easily. The eyes may be affected, with clouding of the lens (cataract) and loss of vision due to nerve damage (optic atrophy). Loss of hearing may also occur due to nerve damage. Premature ageing of the skin is common, with wrinkles developing on the face, legs and arms. This is due to a loss of fat from beneath the skin (subcutaneous adipose tissue). Individuals with this disease may have more pigmentation in their skin and may have pale brown patches on the skin, known as café-au-lait spots. Other symptoms include diminished or weakened reflexes (hyporeflexia), developmental delay and behavioural problems, inability to control involuntary movements (ataxia), feeding difficulties in infancy, dental abnormalities, a clubbed foot, high muscle tone (hypertonia), spine abnormalities and restricted joint movements. Characteristic facial features include an abnormally small head, a face with a pinched appearance, deep-set eyes, a beaked nose and a projecting jaw (prognathism). The symptoms of Cockayne syndrome develop gradually over a number of years. Vision, hearing and functioning of the nervous system worsen over time.

This disorder can be diagnosed on the basis of a range of routine tests designed to eliminate other disorders. Other tests may include a skeletal radiograph, a CT scan, an electroencephalogram, an electroretinogram and cultured skin biopsy analysis. Treatment of this disorder aims to relieve any symptoms and provide support in the care of the individual. This may include specialist education, physical therapy, and consultations with skin specialists as well as eye and hearing specialists. As children with Cockayne syndrome are sensitive to ultraviolet light, extra care will need to be taken to provide them with extra protection from sunlight. The severity of the disorder in children varies, but few survive beyond midlife. Genetic counselling may be of benefit to those affected by this disorder.

Reviewed by Dr RE Pugh

Drash syndrome

Other names for this condition

- DDS
- Denys–Drash syndrome
- Nephropathy–pseudohermaphroditism–Wilms' tumour
- Pseudohermaphroditism–nephron disorder–Wilms' tumour
- Wilms' tumour and pseudohermaphroditism
- Wilms' tumour–pseudohermaphroditism–nephropathy
- Wilms' tumour–pseuodohermaphroditism–glomerulopathy

Drash syndrome is a rare disorder that mainly affects males. It is characterised by abnormal kidney function, a cancerous tumour of the kidney known as Wilms' tumour, and genital abnormalities. Those who have the incomplete form of the disorder show abnormal kidney function with either Wilms' tumour or genital abnormalities. This disorder is thought to be mainly due to mutations in the Wilms' tumour suppressor gene (*WT1*), which is located on the short arm of chromosome 11.

Drash syndrome mostly occurs sporadically for no reason, although in rare cases it is inherited in an autosomal dominant manner.

Symptoms of this disorder include progressive kidney disease (often leading to kidney failure during the first 3 years of life) and Wilms' tumour, which is the commonest form of childhood kidney cancer. This can be detected by poor appetite, abdominal pain and swelling, a hernia protruding through the abdominal wall, blood in the urine, fever, pallor and/or lethargy. Male pseudohermaphroditism is also a major symptom. This is characterised by incomplete development of the testes and external sexual organs, which are either not identifiable as entirely male or female, or are completely female. These males may not develop external sexual organs until puberty. Individuals affected by Drash syndrome may develop malignancies of the testes or ovaries. Screening of these areas will determine this. Some patients may develop a blockage in the tubes that carry urine from the kidney to the bladder, causing a backflow of urine from the bladder (hydronephrosis).

Treatment of Drash syndrome depends mainly on the symptoms of the disorder, although patients with progressive kidney failure can be maintained on dialysis. In this case, toxins that would normally be excreted from the body in the urine are instead removed from the blood by a machine. Some patients may have their kidneys removed (bilateral nephrectomy) and then go on to have renal replacement therapy. Those affected may also have their testes or ovaries removed to reduce the risk of malignancy. Other treatment may include management of fluid and electrolytes, treatment for high blood pressure, and chemotherapy for patients with Wilms' tumour. Genetic counselling is recommended for those affected by this condition.

Reviewed by Professor PM Stewart

Hallervorden–Spatz syndrome

Other names for this condition

- HSD
- Neurodegeneration with brain iron accumulation type 1 (NBIA1)
- Neuroaxonal dystrophy, late infantile
- Pantothenate kinase-associated neurodegeneration

In this rare disorder there is a progressive degeneration of the nervous system, frequently associated with an accumulation of iron in certain areas of the brain. There are two forms of the disorder – a classical form and an atypical form. In the classical form there is a deficiency or an absence of the enzyme pantothenate kinase, due to mutations in the *PANK2* gene.

The pattern of inheritance for this disorder is autosomal recessive.

Symptoms commonly appear during the first 10 years of life, and usually affect motor development, with frequent falls and difficulty in walking, which can appear as clumsiness. As the condition progresses, over a period of 10–15 years there is increasing muscle rigidity, which eventually leads to loss of the ability to walk and move. There may be sudden involuntary muscle spasms (choreoathetosis) with repetitive movements and unusual postures, or an abnormality in muscle tone (dystonia) that can lead to prolonged contraction of muscles.

As the muscles of the mouth and throat become involved, speech and swallowing problems develop. There may be a loss of clarity of speech and word formation (dysarthria), and an inability to say a word that is in the mind (dysphasia). Difficulty in swallowing (dysphagia) is common. Over time, normal eating becomes too difficult and tube or gastrostomy feeding is needed. Inability to swallow saliva also leads to excessive drooling. Impairment of the eyesight is not uncommon, and this may be caused by either degeneration of the retina due to an excess of pigmentation (retinitis pigmentosa), or involvement of the optic nerve (optic atrophy). Progressive intellectual impairment (dementia) is common, and some individuals have seizures. Over time, there is an inexorable deterioration, with loss of skills and functions. However, affected individuals may remain stable for long periods, which are interspersed with periods of rapid change. The severity of the symptoms and the rate of progression may vary widely from one individual to another.

In the atypical form of the disorder, the genetic alterations that lead to the condition have not yet been identified, and the methods of inheritance are unclear. The symptoms of this form usually develop later, around adolescence, and progress more slowly than those of the classical form. The symptoms that are more likely to present first are speech problems, including loss of the ability to speak clearly and form words (dysarthria), repetition of words or phrases (palilalia) and speaking rapidly (tachylalia). There may be changes in behaviour, such as mood swings, depression, impulsive behaviour and violent outbursts. As the condition progresses, the movement problems seen in the classical form develop, with difficulty in controlling movements and eventually loss of the ability to walk. Seizures are more likely to occur in the atypical form. The symptoms in this form of Hallervorden–Spatz syndrome show greater variation between individuals.

Treatment for those with both classical and atypical forms of Hallervorden–Spatz syndrome aims to relieve any symptoms and provide support in the care of the individual. Physical therapy and speech therapy are often of benefit. Various drugs can help to ameliorate the abnormalities in muscle tone, movement and drooling. Botulinum injections can relieve some muscle spasms, and anti-epileptic drugs can help to prevent seizures if they are present. Unfortunately, however, at present there is no specific treatment for the disease itself.

Reviewed by Dr M Webster

Menkes disease

Other names for this condition
- Copper transport disease
- Kinky hair disease
- Steely hair disease
- Trichopoliodystrophy
- X-linked copper deficiency
- X-linked copper malabsorption

This disorder affects the body's ability to use copper, which results in an abnormal accumulation of copper in the liver. As the copper is not being processed, this leads to a deficiency in most of the body's tissues, including the hair, brain, bones, liver and arteries. Most affected individuals present with a classical severe form, although some individuals have milder forms. The form is dependent on the level of copper deficiency.

This disorder is inherited in an X-linked manner.

The characteristic symptom is sparse, steely or 'kinky' hair that is easily broken and is often white or grey in colour. There may be unusual facial features, including chubby cheeks and a broad depressed nasal bridge. Affected individuals are often born prematurely, and symptoms of the condition usually appear during infancy. Common symptoms include lower than normal body temperature (hypothermia), raised levels of bilirubin in the blood (hyperbilirubinaemia), which may cause yellowing of the skin and eyes (jaundice), a delay in physical and mental development (developmental delay), failure to grow and gain weight (failure to thrive), a lack of muscle tone (hypotonia), a loss of previously acquired skills, and fits (seizures). In some individuals there may be blood clots or ruptures of arteries in the brain, as well as weakening of the bones (osteoporosis) that can result in fractures. The severity of the symptoms varies from one individual to another depending on the level of deficiency. In the classical severe form individuals rarely survive beyond 3 years of age.

This disorder may be diagnosed on the basis of a clinical evaluation, blood tests, skin biopsy, microscopic hair examination and biopsy of the placenta to show copper abnormalities. Treatment aims to relieve any symptoms and provide support in the care of the individual. Physiotherapy may be of benefit, and a high-calorie diet is recommended. Intramuscular copper injections may be of benefit if given in the early stages of the disease. Milder forms of the disorder seem to be associated with more positive results than the severe forms.

Reviewed by Dr RE Pugh

Pelizaeus–Merzbacher disease

Other names for this condition

- PMD
- Pelizaeus–Merzbacher disease
- Pelizaeus–Merzbacher brain sclerosis
- Sclerosis, diffuse familial brain
- Sudanophilic leukodystrophy, Pelizaeus–Merzbacher type

This disorder is characterised by abnormalities of the brain's white matter that affect the central nervous system. There is a lack of fatty coverings (myelin sheaths) on the nerve fibres in the brain. The disorder is caused by an alteration in the gene that controls the production of proteolipid protein (PLP), which is the main protein present within myelin in the brain. There is considerable confusion about the use of the term 'Pelizaeus–Merzbacher disease' in the literature.

It is currently deemed desirable to reserve the designation Pelizaeus–Merzbacher disease for the disorder due to abnormality of PLP, a disorder inherited as an X-linked recessive trait. Classically this presents in late infancy, although some reported cases have presented in the neonatal period, or in early infancy, and have therefore been termed the connatal form. There is a separate autosomal recessive disorder that can mimic the connatal form, although the majority of connatal cases are X-linked. Similarly, an autosomal recessive disorder has been described with mutations in the *GJA12* gene that is said to be 'Pelizaeus–Merzbacher-like.'

An adult-onset disorder that resembles multiple sclerosis and follows autosomal dominant inheritance has also been termed 'late-onset Pelizaeus–Merzbacher disease', but is clearly a separate entity due to mutations in a completely different gene.

Classical Pelizaeus–Merzbacher disease is an X-linked disorder.

The symptoms of this disease appear slowly but are progressive, and can vary from one individual to another. The classical form of this disease usually begins in infancy. Early symptoms include feeding difficulties, an inability to control the head, and rapid eye movements (nystagmus) that may not be recognised until several months of age. In rare cases, nystagmus does not develop. Nystagmus may disappear with age. These children have floppy muscles (hypotonia) and develop a tremor of the head and neck, ataxia (unsteadiness) and spastic quadriparesis (stiffness of the arms and legs) beginning in the first five years. They usually have some voluntary control of their arms. If walking skill is acquired, it usually requires crutches or a walker, and is lost as spasticity increases during later childhood or adolescence. Cognitive abilities are impaired, but language and speech usually develop. Extrapyramidal abnormalities, such as dystonic posturing and athetosis, may occur. Survival into the sixth or seventh decade has been observed.

In the connatal form of the disorder, symptoms start to appear during the first few weeks of life, and include weakness, physical and mental abnormalities, failure to reach developmental milestones, and repeated episodes of vomiting that may progress to projectile vomiting. This form of the disorder is more severe and progresses more quickly than the classical form.

Some faults in the PLP gene have not resulted in the clinical picture of Pelizaeus–Merzbacher disease, but instead cause a milder condition with spasticity of the legs but little or no cognitive impairment and a normal lifespan.

Pelizaeus–Merzbacher disease can be diagnosed on the basis of clinical evaluation, a detailed family history and a range of specialist tests, including an MRI scan of the brain (which shows very delayed or even absent myelination) and a search for an alteration in the PLP gene (which may be either a duplication of the gene or a fault within the gene itself).

Treatment for this condition is symptomatic and supportive. It aims to relieve symptoms and make the individual as comfortable as possible. For example, medications can be given to prevent seizures and to ease movement disorders. This condition is progressively terminal in most cases, although the speed of progression and the prognosis vary from one individual to another. Genetic counselling for those affected is recommended.

Reviewed by Dr A Fryer

Reye syndrome

Other names for this condition
- Fatty liver with encephalopathy
- RS

Reye syndrome is a rare disorder that affects all of the organs, but is mainly characterised by fatty changes in the liver and sudden swelling of the brain (cerebral oedema). It most commonly affects people aged around 4 to 18 years. In rare instances, young infants or adults may be affected.

The cause of Reye syndrome is unknown, although it is believed that the disorder may be associated with the use of aspirin-containing medicines to treat chickenpox or flu in children. It may also be linked with other infections, such as rubella, influenza A, herpes simplex or Epstein–Barr syndrome. Some researchers have suggested that the disorder is caused by abnormal functioning of the cell structures that break down sugars, fatty acids and carbohydrates to provide energy (mitochondria), and that the liver mitochondrial enzymes show reduced activity. Some metabolic disorders may have symptoms that resemble those that are associated with Reye syndrome.

Symptoms of this disorder usually present approximately 5 to 7 days following an infection. They may vary in severity, and may or may not be progressive. Symptoms include persistent vomiting, loss of consciousness, irritability, lethargy, disorientation and restlessness. Some individuals may develop memory loss and become unaware of their surroundings. Other symptoms include dilated pupils, breathing abnormalities, a rapid heartbeat, reduced or absent reflexes, seizures, an abnormal posture, jaundice, an enlarged liver (hepatomegaly), an increased level of liver enzymes known as hepatic transaminases, and high levels of ammonia in the blood.

This disorder is diagnosed on the basis of a patient's medical history, physical examination and clinical tests, including liver function tests and blood tests. Reye syndrome should be suspected in any child with unexplained acute swelling of the brain and severe vomiting. This disorder may be misdiagnosed as any disease that impairs the functioning of the brain (encephalopathy), meningitis, diabetes, drug overdose, poisoning, psychiatric illness or sudden infant death syndrome (SIDS). Treatment of Reye syndrome aims to relieve any symptoms and provide support in the care of the individual. Treatment is primarily based on preventing permanent damage to the brain as a result of swelling. Affected individuals may need intensive care and close observation. Fluids with electrolytes and glucose may be administered intravenously, and a respirator may be needed to aid breathing. Medications may be used to control swelling of the brain and to remove ammonia from the blood. Genetic counselling may be of benefit to those affected by this disorder.

Reviewed by Dr A Chakrapani

Smith–Lemli–Opitz syndrome

Other names for this condition
- 7-dehydrocholesterol reductase deficiency
- RHS syndrome
- SLO syndrome
- SLOS
- Smith–Opitz inborn syndrome

In this disorder there is an absence or a deficiency of the enzyme 7-dehydrocholesterol reductase. This is needed to convert 7-dehydrocholesterol into cholesterol. Cholesterol is required when an embryo is developing, and also for optimal growth and brain development after birth.

This disorder is genetically inherited from the parents in an autosomal recessive manner.

The onset of symptoms begins before birth, and the range and severity of symptoms vary from one individual to another. Some individuals may only have one or two symptoms, whereas others may have most of the symptoms described below. In this disorder, symptoms may include a low birth weight, failure to grow and gain weight, a delay in physical and mental development, vomiting, a shrill cry, a small head (microcephaly) that is long and narrow, a horizontal crease across the palms of the hands and the soles of the feet, and drooping eyelids (blepharoptosis).

Other symptoms of this disorder include a broad nose tip, low-set ears, a small jaw (micrognathia), webbing between the second and third toes, an extra finger or toe (polydactyly), a failure of the roof of the mouth to join in the middle (cleft palate), feeding difficulties, a narrowing of the outlet from the stomach (pyloric stenosis), mild to severe learning difficulties and behavioural problems. There may be a failure of the testes to descend in males, the urethra may open on the underside of the penis (hypospadias) and the penis may be small in size. In some individuals, the heart, lungs, liver and kidneys may also be affected.

Treatment for individuals with this disease aims to relieve any symptoms and provide support in the care of the individual. It is thought that supplements of natural cholesterol, such as egg yolk, meat and cream, or purified cholesterol may aid the growth and development of affected individuals. It should be noted that breast milk is rich in cholesterol, unlike formula milks, but still will not provide sufficient for a baby's requirements. If feeding problems are severe, tube feeding may be helpful. Surgery may be necessary if pyloric stenosis or cleft palate is present. Treatment may also be required if the heart, lungs, liver or kidneys are affected. Physical therapy and educational support can also be of benefit.

Reviewed by Professor M Gardiner

Timothy syndrome

Other names for this condition
- Long QT syndrome with syndactyly

Timothy syndrome is a rare disorder caused by alterations in one of the calcium-channel genes. Calcium channels regulate how much calcium can enter a cell. When these channels are defective, the cells become overwhelmed by an influx of calcium. The calcium channel related to Timothy syndrome is known as the CaV1.2 channel. This disorder is caused by a defect in the *CACNA1C* gene, which is located on the short arm of chromosome 12 (12p13.3).

In the majority of cases, Timothy syndrome is caused by a spontaneous defect in the *CACNA1C* gene. However, there has been one family reported with two affected children. For further information, a genetic counselling service should be consulted.

Symptoms of this disorder include webbing (syndactyly) of the hands and feet, intermittent hypoglycaemia, a weakened immune system, baldness at birth, a flat nasal bridge, a small upper jaw, low-set ears and small and/or misplaced teeth. Children with Timothy syndrome may have deficits in language and social development, and some children may also have a form of autism.

Problems with the heart rhythm (arrhythmias) are the most serious aspect of Timothy syndrome, and many affected children suffer life-threatening collapses. These heart rhythm problems are associated with an abnormality on the ECG known as a long QT interval. Structural heart defects are also symptoms of this disorder. These include a cardiovascular defect caused by the failure of the arterial canal to close after birth (patent ductus arteriosus). In addition, there is a complex congenital heart defect that occurs between the time shortly after conception and the end of the second month of pregnancy. It causes reduced blood flow to the lungs, mixing of oxygenated and deoxygenated blood inside the heart, and low levels of oxygen in the blood, leading to cyanosis and a bluish discoloration of the skin (tetralogy of Fallot). Membranous ventricular septal defect is a congenital heart abnormality that is caused by the failure of the muscular portion of the wall separating the lower chambers of the heart (the interventricular septum) to fuse with the free edge of the portion that separates the tricuspid and pulmonary valves in the heart (conus septum). The average lifespan of affected individuals is 2.5 years, and females appear to have a higher survival rate than males. The oldest known living individual with Timothy syndrome is 20 years old.

Diagnosis of this condition is made after children born with webbed fingers and toes (syndactyly) are automatically checked to see whether they have a genetic disorder. An electrocardiogram and an echocardiogram will detect heart defects that would point towards a diagnosis of Timothy syndrome. Autism is a complex disorder and may be more difficult to detect. Researchers are treating these children with calcium-channel-blocking drugs in the hope that these medications will reduce irregular heart rhythms and improve cognitive function.

Research into how calcium-channel-blocking drugs affect individuals with this disorder and how abnormal calcium flow may be related to autism is ongoing.

Reviewed by Dr A Fryer

Xeroderma pigmentosum

Other names for this condition

- XP

This is a group of disorders that is characterised by extreme sensitivity to ultraviolet light. The sun is the main source of ultraviolet light. In this group of disorders there is a decrease in the ability of the cells to repair damage to their DNA after exposure to ultraviolet light. This process is called nucleotide excision repair. Each type of XP has a different defect in the repair process.

This disorder is genetically inherited from the parents in an autosomal recessive manner.

Symptoms usually appear in the first few years after birth. However, some individuals may not develop symptoms until later in childhood. The initial symptoms are often excessive freckling and a heightened reaction to the sun (photosensitivity) that causes redness, inflammation, blistering and pain on exposure to the sun. There may also be extreme sensitivity of the eyes to light (photophobia), inflammation of the membranes of the inside of the eyelids and the whites of the eyes (conjunctivitis), inflammation of the cornea (keratitis), excessive watering of the eyes, and clouding of the lens of the eye. Other signs may include darkening of the skin (hyper-pigmentation), diminished pigmentation of the skin (hypopigmentation) and the development of small red skin lesions (telangiectasias) that are caused by widening of blood vessels.

Affected individuals are more susceptible to developing various non-cancerous (benign) and cancerous (malignant) tumours. These include skin cancers induced by exposure to sunlight, such as malignant melanoma, basal-cell carcinoma and squamous-cell carcinoma, which often affect the head, face and neck, and non-cancerous skin tumours (benign) of blood vessels or certain cells, as well as tumours of the eyelid, cornea and the tip of the tongue. In some cases there may be neurological symptoms that can include a delay in mental development, weakened or absent reflexes, a small-sized head (microcephaly), hearing impairment (senso-rineural deafness), increased muscle tension and rigidity, and a loss of the ability to coordinate muscle movements (ataxia). These symptoms are progressive – in other words, they gradually become more severe.

Exposure to the sun should be avoided, in order to protect the skin. If sun exposure cannot be avoided, it must be kept to a minimum, and protection such as double-layering of clothes, a hat, dark glasses and sun cream with an SRF factor of 50 should be used. Ultraviolet-resistant face visors are also available, and are strongly recommended. Windows can be coated with ultraviolet-resistant film to prevent exposure to sunlight, and low-wattage incandescent lighting (using an artificial filament) should be used because of the sensitivity of the eyes to bright lights. Some affected individuals reverse their sleeping pattern so that they sleep during the day and are active at night, to try to avoid sun exposure. If seizures occur, medication may be required. Affected individuals should be regularly monitored by a skin specialist (dermatologist) and an eye specialist (ophthalmologist) to ensure early detection of any skin lesions or eye abnormalities.

Early surgical removal and/or other treatment is required for tumours. It is also important to avoid exposure to other known carcinogens, such as cigarette smoke.

In the past, this disorder has led to a reduced life expectancy due to the susceptibility to development of tumours. However, if an affected child is well protected from sunlight from an early age, and monitored by a dermatologist, a normal lifespan can now be expected. However, if the patient has the disorder with neurological complications, there will be a reduced life expectancy.

Reviewed by Professor AR Lehmann

Index

ABCD1 protein 38
N-acetylaspartic acid 20
N-acetylglutamate synthetase 1
acid beta-glucosidase deficiency 62–3
acid sphingomyelinase (ASM) 68
acrodermatitis enteropathica (AE) 128
acroparasaesthesiae 55
ACTH (adrenocorticotrophic hormone) 96
    deficiency disorders 98
acute intermittent porphyria (AIP) 84
ACY2 (aminoacylase-2) deficiency 20–1
Addison-Schilder disease 38
adenosine deaminase (ADA) deficiency 85
adenosine monophosphate (AMP)
        deaminase deficiency 90
adenylosuccinate lyase deficiency 86
adenylosuccinic acid (AMPS) 86
'adrenal crises' 104
adrenal glands 96
adrenaline 96
adrenocorticotrophic hormone (ACTH) 96
    deficiency disorders 98
adrenoleukodystrophy (ALD) – X-linked
    38–9
adrenomyeloneuropathy (AMN) 38–9
ADSL deficiency 86
alaninuria 51–2
Albright hereditary osteodystrophy (AHO)
    99–100
aldehyde oxidase deficiencies 10, 95
aldosterone 96
Aldrich syndrome 141–2
alfacalcidol 126
alkaline phosphatase 128
Alper's disease 40–1
alpha-1-antitrypsin deficiency (A1AD)
    129–30
alpha-galactosidase A deficiency 55–6
alpha-L-fucosidase deficiency 60–1
amaurotic familial idiocy 69
Amicar® 139–40
amino acid disorders, general characteristics
    1
aminoacylase-2 deficiency 20–1
aminolevulinic acid (ALA) 84

ammonia metabolism 1
    see also hyperammonaemic episodes
amniocentesis 31, 33
amylo-1, 6-glucosidase deficiency 78
amyloidosis, general characteristics 111
Anderson-Fabry disease 55–6
angiohaemophilia 139–40
angiokeratoma corporis diffusum 55–6
angiokeratomas 55, 60
anidiuretic hormone (ADH) 96
antitrypsin deficiency 129–30
aplastic anaemia 50
apoplipoprotein AI/II amyloidosis 111
arginase deficiencies 1
arginine 3, 4, 13
argininosuccinase aciduria (ASA) 2–3
argininosuccinate lyase (ASL) 1
    deficiency disorders 2–3
argininosuccinate synthetase (ASS) 1
    deficiency disorders 4
ASA (argininosuccinase aciduria) 2–3
Ashkenazi Jewish descendants 68, 69, 144
ASL (argininosuccinate lyase) 1
    deficiency disorders 2–3
aspartoacylase (ASP) deficiency 20–1
ASS (argininosuccinate synthetase) 1
    deficiency disorders 4
ataxia telangiectasia (AT) 131–2
ATM gene 131
autoimmune disorders, general
        characteristics 127, 141
autosomal dominant inheritance xi
autosomal recessive inheritance xi

Babinski sign 64
Bannayan-Riley-Ruvalcaba syndrome
        (BRRS) 101–2
Barth syndrome 28–9
Batten disease-infantile form 57
BCKD deficiency 8–9
Bean syndrome 133
behavioural counselling 35
Berardinelli-Seip lipodystophy 65
bile acid precursors 37
bilirubin-UGT 135

biotin 34
biotinidase deficiency 103
blood disorders, general characteristics 127
Bloom syndrome 144
blue rubber bleb naevus syndrome 133
bone marrow disorders, Pearson's syndrome 50
bone-marrow transplants 39, 61, 62–3, 85, 91, 142
Bonnevie-Ulrich syndrome 137–8
botulinum injections 149
bovine ADA 85
Bowen syndrome 53
branched-chain alpha-ketoacid dehydrogenase deficiency 8–9
Brandt syndrome 128
BRBNS 133
British Porphyria Association 84, 93
Bronze Schilder's disease 38–9
BRRS (Bannayan-Riley-Ruvalcaba syndrome) 101–2
Brunzell syndrome 65
BZS (Bannayan-Zonana syndrome) 101–2

CACNA1C gene 155
CAH (congenital adrenal hyperplasia) disorders 104
calcitriol 126
calcium channel genes 155
calcium regulation 96, 155
   disorders 99–100, 126
calcium supplementation 126
Canavan leukodystrophy 20–1
carbamyl phosphate synthetase 1
carbohydrate disorders, general characteristics 70
carbohydrate-reduced diets 45, 52, 77
cardiac transplants 29
cardiolipin 28
cardioskeletal myopathy with neutropenia and abnormal mitochondria 28–9
carnitine palmitoyltransferase (CPT) deficiency 22–3
carnitine supplements 35
   specific disorders 22–3, 24, 27, 31, 32, 41
cataracts
   galactokinase deficiencies 75
   Lowe syndrome 121–2
Cbl disorders 30–1
CD 20–1
ceramide trihexosidase deficiency 55–6

cerebello-oculocutaneous telangiectasia 131–2
cerebrohepatorenal syndrome 53
cerebromacular degeneration 69
Ceredase® 62
Cerezyme® 62
Charcot-Marie-Tooth (CMT) disease 112–13
cholesterol disorders, general characteristics 54, 154
cholesterol-rich diets 154
choline
   food sources 35
   metabolism 35
chorionic villus sampling (CVS) 20, 31, 33
Christensen's disease 40–1
chronic progressive external ophthalmoplegia with myopathy 43
citrullinaemia 4
citrulline supplementation 13
classical galactosaemia 75–6
cleft palate, velocardiofacial syndrome 124–5
CLIMB (Children Living with Inherited Metabolic Diseases) x
cobalamin (Cbl) metabolism disorders 30–1
cochlear implants 47
Cockayne syndrome 145–6
coenzyme Q10 41, 47, 52
Coffin-Lowry syndrome (CLS) 114–15
Coffin-Siris syndrome 103
combined uraciluria-thyminuria 87
complex IV deficiency 48–9
congenital adrenal hyperplasia (CAH) disorders 104
congenital adrenal hyperplasia-3-beta-hydroxysteroid dehydrogenase 104
congenital disorders of glycosylation (CDGs), general characteristics 70
congenital disorders of glycosylation-type 1a 71–2
congenital generalised lipodystrophy 65
congenital hyperinsulinism 80
congenital infantile lactic acidosis 51–2
congenital sucrose intolerance 81
congenital tyrosinosis 17–18
connective tissue disorders, general characteristics 110
constitutional liver dysfunction 135
constitutional thrombopathy 139–40
copper transport disease 150
Cori disease 78
cornstarch 78, 79

corticotrophin 96
cortisol 96
cortisol replacement therapy 104
Cowden/Bannayan-Riley-Ruvalcaba overlap
    syndrome 101–2
COX deficiencies 48–9
CPEO with myopathy 43
cryoprecipitate 140
cryptorchidism-drawfism-subnormal
    mentality 108–9
CSID 81
Cyklokapron® 139–40
Cystagon® 59
cystathionine beta-synthase (CBS) 7
cystatin C amyloidosis 111
Cysteamine 59
cystinosis 58–9
cytochrome C oxidase deficiency 48–9

Danbolt-Cross syndrome 128
Dandy-Walker syndrome 103
DDS 147
De Toni-Fanconi-Debré syndrome 48–9
De Vivo disease 77
deafness-dwarfism-retinal atrophy 145–6
debrancher deficiency 78
deficiency of electron transfer flavoprotein
    32
7-dehydrocholesterol reductase deficiency
    154
Denys-Drash syndrome 147
dextromethorphan 12
diabetes mellitus 65
    and hyperinsulinism-hypoglycaemia 80
dialysis 31
diazepam 12
dicarboxylic aminoaciduria 24–5
diffuse cerebral degeneration in infancy
    40–1
DiGeorge syndrome 124–5
dihydropyrimidine dehydrogenase deficiency
    87
dihydroxycholestanoic acid 37
diodoquin 128
disaccharide intolerance I 81
disorders of *N*-glycan processing-type 1a
    71–2
DNA testing
    epidermolysis bullosa 117
    fructoseaemia 74
Donohue syndrome 107
Dowling-Meara EB variants 116–17

Drash syndrome 147
dwarfism with renal atrophy and deafness
    145–6
dwarfism-onychodysplasia 103
dysostosis multiplex 54

electron transfer flavoprotein (ETF) enzyme
    32
encephalitis periaxialis diffusa 38–9
endocardial fibroelastosis type-2 28–9
enzyme replacement therapies 12, 56, 61,
    62–3, 67, 81
epidermolysis bullosa (EB) 116–17
EPM2 120
ETF-QO enzyme 32

Fabrazyme® 56
Fabry crises 55
Fabry disease 55–6
factor X deficiency 134
familial amyloidotic polyneuropathy 111
familial chronic obstructive lung disease
    129–30
familial emphysema 129–30
familial hyperinsulinism 80
Fanconi syndrome 17
Fanconi II syndrome 58–9
Fanconi-Bickel syndrome 73
fatty acid oxidation disorders, general
    characteristics 19
fatty liver with encephalopathy 153
favism 136
fibrinogen amyloidosis 111
fibroblastic growth factor-23 (FGF23) 126
fifth-digit syndrome 103
FISH (fluorescence *in-situ* hybridisation)
    analysis 124
fish odour syndrome 35–6
5-fluorouracil 87
Flatau-Schilder disease 38–9
flavin-containing monooxygenase-2 35–6
fludrocortisone 104
FMO2 35–6
follicle-stimulating hormone (FSH) 96
45, X syndrome 137–8
fructosaemia 74
fructose intolerance-hereditary 74
FUCA1 gene 60
fucosidosis 60–1
Fuller-Albright syndrome-1 99–100
fumarase deficiency 42
fumarylacetoacetase deficiency 17–18

G6PF deficiency 136
galactokinase deficiency 75, 82
galactosaemia 75–6
galactose-free diets 76, 82
GALE (uridine diphosphate galactose-4-
    epimerase) deficiency 82
GALT (galactose-1-phosphate uridyl
    transferase) deficiencies 75–6, 82
gangliosidosis hexosaminidase deficiencies
    64, 69
gas chromatography-mass spectrometry 20
Gaucher disease type-1 62–3
GBA deficiency 62–3
gelsolin amyloidosis 111
gene therapies 142
Gilbert syndrome 135
GJA12 gene 151
GLA deficiency 55–6
glucocerebrosidase deficiency 62–3
glucose administration 2–3, 4, 13, 80, 84,
    93
glucose transporter type 1 deficiency 77
glucose-6-phosphate dehydrogenase
    deficiency 136
GLUT1 gene 77
GLUT2 gene 73
glutaric aciduria (GA) type-1 24–5
glutaric aciduria (GA) type-II 32
glutaryl-CoA dehydrogenase deficiency
    24–5
glycine accumulation disorders 11–12,
    30–1, 33–4
glycine encepephalopathy 11–12
glycine supplementation 26, 32
glycogen storage diseases
    type O 79
    type III 78
    type XI 73
glycogen synthase deficiency 79
glycogenosis
    Fanconi type 73
    type O 79
    type III 78
glycoprotein functions 71
glycosylation disorders, general
    characteristics 70
GM2 gangliosidosis type-1 69
GM2 gangliosidosis type-2 infantile form 64
gonadal dysgenesis 137–8
gonadotrophins 96
granulocyte-colony stimulating factor (G-
    CSF) 29

GROD (granular osmiophilic deposits) 57
growth hormones 96
    deficiency disorders 105
    replacement therapies 122, 138

haem arginate 84, 93
Hallervorden-Spatz syndrome 148–9
haloperidol 88
hamartomas 101–2
Hart syndrome 5–6
Hartnup disease 5–6
heel prick (PKU) test 1, 15
hepatatorenal tyrosinaemia 17–18
hepatorenal glycogenosis with renal
    Fanconi syndrome 73
hereditary emphysema 129–30
hereditary fructose intolerance (HFI) 74
hereditary hyperuricaemia and
    choreoathetosis syndrome 88–9
hereditary motor and sensory neuropathy
    (HMSN) 112–13
hereditary nephropathic amyloidosis 111
hereditary renal amyloidosis 111
hereditary xanthinuria 95
hexosaminidase deficiencies 64
high-fat diets
    Leigh syndrome 45
    pyruvate dehydrogenase deficiency 52
hirsutism 65
HND see Hartnup disease
homocysteinaemia 7
homocystinuria 7
hormone disorders, general characteristics
    96
HPRT, absence of 88
3ß-HSD 104
Humatrope 138
Hunter disease 66–7
Hutchinson-Gilford progeria syndrome
    (HGPS) 118–19
hydrocortisone supplementation 104
hyperammonaemia type-II 13–14
hyperammonaemic episodes
    described 1
    metabolic conditions 2–3, 4, 13–14
    treatments 2–3
hyperbilirubinaemia-I 135
hypergalactosaemia 73
hyperglycinaemia with ketoacidosis and
    lactic acidosis 33–4
hyperinsulinism-hypoglycaemia 80
hyperphenylalaninaemia 15–16

hyperplasia 104
hyperuricaemia-oligophrenia 88–9
hypogenital dystrophy with diabetic
    tendency 108–9
hypophosphataemic rickets 73
hypopituitarism 106
hypothyroidism 100
hypotonia-hypomentia-hypogonadism-
    obesity syndrome 108–9
hypouricaemia 10
hypoxanthine-guanine
    phosphoribosyltransferase (HGPRT)
    88–9

Icterus intermittens juvenlis 135
iduronate-2-sulphatase deficiency 66–7
IMD2 141–2
immune system disorders, general
    characteristics 127, 141
immunodeficiency with ataxia telangiectasia
    131–2
immunodeficiency with thrombocytopenia
    and eczema 141–2
inborn error of urea synthesis,
    citrullinaemia type-1 4
infantile cerebral ganglioside storage 69
infantile neuronal ceroid lipofuscinosis
    (INCL) 57
insulin control 96
intermittent ataxia with lactic acidosis 51–2
invertase 81
iodoquinol 128
iron accumulations 148
iron supplements 117, 133
Islet dysregulation syndrome 80
isoleucine 8–9, 30
isovaleric acidaemia (IVA) 26

junctional epidermolysis bullosa (JEB) 116
juvenile gout, choreoathetosis and mental
    retardation syndrome 88–9

Kearns-Sayre syndrome 43, 50
ketamine 12
ketogenic diets 77
ketonaemia 30–1
ketosis disorders 30–1, 33–4
ketotic glycinaemia 33–4
kinky hair disease 150
Kreb's cycle disorders 42

L-carnitine supplements 35

specific disorders 23, 24, 27, 31, 32, 41
L-cycloserine 63
lactic acidosis 46, 48, 51
    treatments 52
lactic and pyruvate acidaemia with
    carbohydrate sensitivity 51–2
lactose-free diets 76
Lafora body disease 120
Leigh syndrome 44–5, 48–9, 51
leprechaunism 107
Lesch-Nyhan disease 88–9
leucine 8–9, 26
leucine-restricted diets 26
light sensitivity 58
    Bloom syndrome 144
    Cockayne syndrome 145–6
    Hartnup disease 5–6
    variegate porphyria 93–4
    xeroderma pigmentosum (XP) 157–8
lignac-Fanconi syndrome 58–9
limit dextrinosis 78
lipid disorders, general characteristics 54
lipidosis ganglioside infantile 69
lipidosis sphingomyelin 68
lipoatrophic diabetes 65
lipodystrophy-Berardinelli-Seip syndrome 65
lipoic acid supplements 52
lissencephaly (smooth brain) 42
liver glycogen synthase deficiency 79
liver transplantations 3, 18, 41
long QT syndrome with syndactyly 155–6
Lorenzo's oil 39
Louis-Bar syndrome 131–2
low-fat diets, for adrenoleukodystrophy
    (ALD) – X-linked 39
low-protein diets *see* protein restricted diets
Lowe syndrome (LS) 121–2
lung transplants 129–30
luteinising hormone (LH) 96
lysosomal disorders, general characteristics
    54
lysozyme amyloidosis 111

Macrocephaley, multiple lipomas and
    haemangiomata 101
MADD (multiple acyl CoA dehydrogenase
    deficiency) 32
maple syrup disease 8–9
MCADD (medium-chain acyl CoA
    dehydrogenase) deficiency 27
melanodermic leukodystrophy 38–9
MELAS 46–7

Menkes disease 150
metabolic acidosis, treatments 9
metabolic diseases, inheritance routes xi
methionine 7, 30
methylcobalamin deficiency 7
methylene tetrahydrofolate reductase
    deficiency 7
methylglutaconic aciduria (3)-type-2 28–9
methylmalonic acidaemia 7, 30–1
Meulengracht's disease 135
MGA type-II 28–9
Miglustat^R 63, 64
Minot-Von Willebrand disease 139–40
mitochondrial cytopathy (Kearns-Sayre
    type) 43
mitochondrial disorders, general
    characteristics 37
mitochondrial DNA xi
mitochondrial encephalomyopathies,
    general characteristics 43
mitochondrial encephalopathy lactic
    acidosis and stroke-like episodes
    (MELAS) 46–7
mitochondrial enzyme deficiencies 22–3, 27
mitochondrial respiratory chain complex IV
    48–9
molybdenum cofactor deficiency (MOCOD)
    10, 95
monosomy X 137–8
Morgagni-Turner-Albright syndrome 137–8
MtDNA inheritance xi
mucopolusaccharidoses (MPS) 66
mucopolysaccharidosis type-2 66–7
multiple acyl CoA dehydrogenase deficiency
    32
musculoskeletal disorders, general
    characteristics 110
myelinoclastic diffuse sclerosis 38–9
myoadenylate deaminase (MAD) deficiency
    90
myopathy with deficiency of carnitine
    palmitoyltransferase 22–3

N-butyl-dexynojirimycin (NB-DNJ) 63
N-linked oligosaccharides 70
necrotising encephalomyelopathy (of Leigh)
    44–5
Neill-Dingwall syndrome 145
neonatal cholestasis 129–30
neuroaxonal dystrophy, late infantile 148–9
neurodegeneration with brain iron
    accumulation type-1 (NBIA1) 148–9

neuroendocrine glands 96
neutropenia 31
Niemann-Pick disease (NPD)-type A 68
non-ketotic hyperglycinaemia (NKH) 11–12
non-ketotic hypoglycaemia and carnitine
    deficiency 27
Normosang^R 84, 93
NTBC (Nitisinone^R) 18
nucleotide excision repair 157
Nutropin 138

OCRL1 gene 121
oculocerebrorenal syndrome 121–2
oculocraniosomatic neuromuscular disease
    43
oestrogen therapy 138
olivopontocerebellar atrophy 71
opisthotonos 10
opthalmoplegia plus syndrome 43
organic acid disorders, general
    characteristics 19, 30
ornithine transcarbamylase 1
    deficiency disorders 13–14
osteomalacia 126
OTC (ornithine transcarbamylase deficiency)
    13–14
ovarian dwarfism, Turner type 137–8
OXPHOS (oxidative phosphorylation)
    enzyme complexes 45

palmitoyl protein thioesterase (PPT) enzyme
    57
pancreatectomies 80
pancreatic disorders 50, 65, 80
pancreatic nesidioblastosis 80
PANK2 gene 148
pantothenate kinase-associated
    neurodegeneration 148–9
pantothenic acid supplementation 29
parathyroid glands 96
Parkinson's disease 62
PCC (propionyl CoA carboxylase) deficiency
    33–4
PDCD 51–2
PDH (pyruvate dehydrogenase) enzymes
    44–5
    deficiencies 51–2
Pearson's syndrome 50
PEG-ADA 85
Pelizaeus-Merzbacher disease (PMD) 151–2
pellagra-cerebellar ataxia-renal
    aminoaciduria syndrome 5–6

peroneal muscular atrophy 112–13
peroxisomal disorders, general
    characteristics 37
persistent hyperinsulinaemic hypoglycaemia
    of infancy 80
phenylketonuria (PKU) 15–16
    tests 1, 15
PHEX gene 126
PHHI 80
phlebomegaly 65
phosphate therapies 126
phosphomannomutase deficiency 71–2
photophobia 58
    see also light sensitivity
PHP (pseudohypoparathyroidism) 99–100
phytanic acids 37
Pi phenotype ZZ 129–30
pituitary gland 96
pituitary insufficiency 106
PKU *see* phenylketonuria (PKU)
PMM deficiency 71–2
PNDC 40–1
POLG1 gene 40
poliodystrophia cerebri progressiva 40–1
porphobilinogen (PBG) 84
porphyrias, general characteristics 83
Prader-Willi syndrome 108–9
progeria 118–19
progeroid nanism 145–6
progressive cerebral poliodystrophy 40–1
progressive myoclonic epilepsies (PMEs)
    general charactieristics 120
    type-2 120
prolactin 96
prolastin treatments 129–30
propionic acidaemia 33–4
protease inhibitor deficiency 129–30
protein metabolism 1
protein restricted diets
    for argininosuccinase aciduria 2–3
    for carnitine palmitoyltransferase (CPT)
        deficiency 22–3
    for citrullinaemia 4
    for maple syrup disease 9
    for methylmalonic acidaemia 31
    for multiple acyl CoA dehydrogenase
        deficiency 32
    for ornithine transcarbamylase deficiency
        13–14
    for phenylketonuria (PKU) 15–16
    for propionic acidaemia 33
    for tyrosinaemia type-1 17–18

protein-rich diets 117
pseudo-phlorizin diabetes 73
pseudo-pseudohypoparathyroidism (PPHP)
    100
pseudohaemophilia 139–40
pseudohermaphroditism-nephron disorder-
    Wilms' tumour 147
pseudohypoaldosteronism type-1 (PHA-1)
    97
pseudohypoparathyroidism (PHP) 99–100
PTEN hamartoma tumour syndrome 101–2
pterygolymphangiectasia 137–8
purine nucleoside phosphorylase (PNP)
    deficiency 91
purine-rich diets 95
purines 83
pyruvate dehydrogenase deficiency 51–2

renal replacement therapies 147
renal tubular acidosis 73
renal-oculocerebrodystrophy 121–2
Replagal® 56
Reye syndrome 153
riboflavin supplements 32, 47
ribose 90
rickets 126
Riley-Smith syndrome 101–2
RSK2 gene 114–15
Russell-Silver syndrome (RSS) 123
Ruvalcaba-Myhre syndrome 101–2

Sacrosidase 81
SAICAR (succinylaminoimidazole
    carboxamide riboside) 86
salt wasting 97
Sanhoff disease 64
Santavouri disease 57
Schereshevkii-Turner syndrome 137–8
Schilder disease 38–9
sclerosis, diffuse familial brain 151–2
screening tests, amino acid disorders 1
Seip syndrome 65
self-injury behaviours 88–9
serum protease inhibitor deficiency 129–30
severe combined immunodeficiency due to
    adenosine deaminase deficiency 85
short stature-onychodysplasia 103
Shprintzen syndrome 124–5
SI (sucrose isomaltase) deficiency 81
sideroblastic anaemia with marrow-cell
    vacuolisation and exocrine pancreatic
    dysfunction 50

Siewerling-Creutzfeldt disease 38
Silver syndrome 123
SLC2A1 gene 77
SLC9A19 gene 5
Smith-Lemli-Opitz syndrome 154
Smith-Opitz inborn syndrome 154
sodium benzoate 3, 4, 12
sodium bicarbonate 45
sodium phenylbutyrate 3, 4
somatostatin 96
South African porphyria 93–4
sphingolipidosis Tay-Sachs 69
sphingomyelinase deficiency 68
stale fish syndrome 35–6
starch-free diets 81
steely hair disease 150
steroid hormonal disorders, general
    characteristics 54
steroid treatments 38–9, 142
sterol disorders, general characteristics 54
strychnine treatments 11–12
Stuart-Prower deficiency 134
subacute necrotising encephalomyelopathy
    (SNE) 44–5
succinylacetone 17
succinylpurinemic autism 86
sucrase isomaltase deficiency 81
sucrose-free diets 81
Sudanophilic leukodystrophies
    adrenoleukodystrophy 38–9
    Pelizaeus-Merzbacher disease 151–2
sulphite oxidase deficiencies 10, 95
sulphite and xanthine oxidase deficiency 10
S-sulphocysteine levels 10
sulphonamide drugs 6
sunlight intolerance
    Bloom syndrome 144
    Cockayne syndrome 145–6
    cystinosis 58–9
    Hartnup disease 5–6
    variegate porphyria 93–4
    xeroderma pigmentosum (XP) 157–8
Swedish porphyria 84

tandem mass spectrometry (TMS) 26
taurine levels 10
Tay-Sachs disease 64
    infantile form 69
thiamine supplementation 9, 52
thiosulphate levels 10
3ß-HSD 104
threonine 30

thrombocytopenia 31
thyroid gland 96
Timothy syndrome 155–6
transthyretin amyloidosis 111
trichopoliodystrophy 150
trihydroxycholestanoic acid 37
trimethylamine
    food sources 35
    metabolism 35
trimethylaminuria syndrome 35–6
tryptophan 5
L-tryptophan ethyl 6
tryptophan pyrrolase deficiency 5–6
Turner syndrome 137–8
22q11 deletion syndrome 124–5
tyrosinaemia type-1 17–18
tyrosine metabolism 17

umbilical cord stem-cell transfusions 142
unconjugated benign bilirubinaemia 135
urea cycle disorders, general characteristics
    1
uric acid deposits 88
uricaciduria 10
uridine diphosphate (UDP) galactose-4-
    epimerase deficiency 75, 82

valine 8–9, 30
Van Bogaert-Bertrand syndrome 20–1
variegate porphyria (VP) 93–4
vascular haemophilia 139–40
velocardiofacial syndrome (VCFS) 124–5
very-long-chain fatty acids (VLCFA) 37
vitamin B1 supplements 9, 52
vitamin B2 supplements 32, 47
vitamin B6 supplements 7
vitamin B12 supplements 31
vitamin C supplements 74
vitamin D supplements 59, 73
vitamin E supplements 132
vitamin K supplements 134
vitamin cofactors 45
Von Willebrand disease (VWD) 139–40

webbed fingers and toes 155–6
Weber-Cockayne EB variants 116
Willebrand-Juergans disease 139–40
Wilms' tumour and pseudohermaphroditism
    147
Wiskott-Adrich syndrome 141–2

X-ALD 38–9

X-linked cardioskeletal myopathy and
  neutropenia 28–9
X-linked copper deficiency 150
X-linked hypophosphataemic rickets 126
X-linked inheritance xi
xanthine oxidase deficiencies 10, 95
XDH deficiency 95

xeroderma pigmentosum (XP) 157–8
XO syndrome 137–8

Zavesca® 63, 64
Zellweger syndrome (ZS) 53
zinc-deficiency, congenital 128